BECOMING A PURPOSE-DRIVEN PHYSICIAN ASSISTANT

RACHEL ALLAIN JURGENSON, MS, PA-C

BECOMING A PURPOSE-DRIVEN PHYSICIAN ASSISTANT

A helpful and entertaining guide
to making the most
of your career

ISBN: 9798579118189
Library of Congress Control Number: 2020924590

Cover design by Rachel Jurgenson

rachellallain@gmail.com

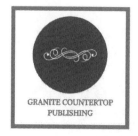

GRANITE COUNTERTOP
PUBLISHING

For You

I have thought about you every moment I have spent on this book.

I want great things for you and your patients.

Table of Contents

Introduction. 1

1. Taking Purpose-Driven First Steps After Graduation. 7

2. Taking Care of Yourself Before You Take Care of Others . . . 19

3. Getting the PA Job You Want. 29

4. Helpful Tips for Working Well With Your
   Attending Physician/Physicians 53

5. Helpful Tips for Working Well With Your Patients 65

6. Helpful Tips for Working Well With Staff Members 89

7. Developing Purposeful Daily Habits and Organizational
   Tips for Success 95

8. Navigating Certification and Recertification 123

9. Managing Difficult Issues 135

10. The Importance of Developing Business Skills
    In Your Practice Setting 145

11. Exploring Additional Pathways
    as a Physician Assistant 153

Post Script. 161

Acknowledgments. 163

Introduction

My first day in a clinical setting, I walked confidently down the hallway at the Houston VA on my way to meet my preceptor. This was the first day they had let us go out into the real world to get some practice on learning how to do a physical exam. Little did I know what practicing medicine had in store for me. Dressed finely in my student length white coat (you know how things work: the shorter the coat, the lowlier the provider, so it might as well had been a halter top I had on) and with all of my handy physical exam tools and accessories at the ready, including my little jar of cinnamon to test the all-important olfactory sensation, I was ready to learn in whatever capacity. As I got to the unit, the nurse at the station informed me my preceptor would be with me in a little bit, which turned out to be about at least thirty minutes later, no surprises there.

When the time came, I met her with all the enthusiasm of a PA student on her first day. I was ready to do a history and physical exam on a real patient, not my fellow students or their cats for that matter (true ophthalmic story). Just point me in the right direction. But, she didn't share my excitement. She looked tired and not all that energetic. "Nice to meet you," she had greeted me. "Come with me. I need to see my next patient."

As I walked into my very first patient's room, the phone was ringing at his bedside and he was not answering. My preceptor picked up the phone, answered it and was observing the patient as she spoke to the person on the other end of the phone.

He was in his bed. He was tall and emaciated, pasty white, with long stringy black hair to his shoulders, and around the age of forty-something. No history was given to me at the time. Apparently there was no time to teach, my goodness, there was barely even time for introductions. I walked further into the room, stood at the foot side of the bed, where his eyes followed and then fixed on me and did not move. All kinds of thoughts and questions were running through my mind, without offering me some sort of answer.

What is going on and why isn't he talking or eager to see me?

Why are his eyes blankly staring at me?

Doesn't he know that he is my very first patient, and I am ready to test his olfactory sensation with my brand-new bottle of cinnamon, and properly identify his diaphragmatic excursion?

"If you want to get down here, you probably should," said my preceptor to the person on the other end of the line. "Ummmh, I think he's dying right now before me." All the while, the patient never took his eyes off me.

What in the world have I gotten myself into? I think, He is not dead, I swear, he is staring right at me. I know when I moved over a little bit, he followed me with his eyes. I can hear him breathing. *Great, I walk in the room; the first patient I see fixes his eyes on me and dies. And why is she just standing there, Call a code green, orange, blue... some color, and let's get out those paddle thingies. I would love to yell 'clear' for the first time, but there's an aching pit in my stomach.*

She hung up the phone, and we stood in silence looking at the gentleman. I was clueless as to what was wrong with the patient, but I could tell is that my preceptor was stressed and exhausted. So, I decided to save my questions for later. At this time, she examines him, he has quit breathing. He is dead. We quietly walk out of the room. He had died of AIDS complications. It is 1996. And, my medical career as a PA is off to a running start! Woo-hoo!

Twenty-four years later, I still work in the medical field and I love being a Physician Assistant. I love working with doctors and patients, and I adore my fellow PAs. I am thankful the majority of patients I come in contact with don't look at me and die. Throughout the years, I have had the opportunity to work in many departments, including gastroenterology, neurosurgery, internal medicine, urgent care, rehab medicine, and cardiology. Most of my time has been in federal service for the VA, but I have also worked for HMOs, a smaller private practice, a locum tenens agency, and a large group of cardiologists. Additionally, I have been an instructor and preceptor at Baylor College of Medicine, and a preceptor for Chicago Medical School (now known as Rosalind Franklin University of Medicine and Science). I have also worked as a law firm consultant and a speaker for St. Jude Medical (now Abbott). More recently, I had the opportunity to work as a clinical specialist for Medtronic and as a technical sales specialist for a diagnostic laboratory company in which I primarily worked within gastroenterology. I have always been in medicine, always teaching, educating, and encouraging patients, their families, providers, and staff.

I am passionate about helping people improve their lives. As providers, you and I teach something every single day. We educate our patients and staff. We are a consultant to our family and friends who call us at any time of day or night. They don't pick up the phone to call their provider—whom they actually pay—because they don't want to wake or bother them. But they never mind calling us and waking us, do they? After all, that's what friends and family are for. Right? Now, if only they would take our advice! But that's an entirely different book or therapy session all-together.

I often get calls from someone who is a friend's cousin's best friend's dad's stepdaughter, asking about what being a PA is like and what exactly it is that I do. I love talking about my experience as a PA, and of course, I have incorporated multiple successful techniques into my PA practice.

Once I graduated, I found that I was just so excited to be done and that I could finally do what I had dreamed of doing, I was done for. Completely done for. It was exhausting going through all of that hard work for two-and-a-half years.

If you are like most PAs, you are a very driven individual. You made an effort to get good grades in high school so that you could go to a great college. And when you got to college, you studied hard to get good grades in all your classes and to get a fabulous score on the GRE, so then you could get to your goal of getting into a PA program. And once you get to PA school, you try to cram everything about medicine into such a short period of time. Then you still set goals of soaking everything in so you can rock the PANCE. Then you knock it out of the park on the PANCE and get that awesome job and you are ready to relax and finally make some money. All this goal setting is exhausting! Aren't we done yet with setting goals and accomplishing them?
My answer to you is NO.

Don't just get out in the medical field and coast for a while. Many PAs can check the box, 'Okay, I am a PA. I'm done,' but I challenge you to not just be an ordinary PA. Be extraordinary! Not just for yourself, but for your patients and their families as well. You have been setting goals all of your life. You have worked extremely hard to get to where you are. You are above coasting. You must continue to strive for excellence by setting both short-term and long-term goals.

There are tons of books out there about being successful in business, relationships, finances, cooking, and sex. However, I find that there is a need for a book that is a quick, fun, and easy tool to help my fellow PAs be purposeful and successful in their career. So whether you have been practicing for many years, just graduated, or you want to know what being a PA is all about, this book is for you.

These are simple but thoughtful practices that I implemented during my many years in medicine. I do not expect everything that works for me to work for you. You will however, learn some simple time-management techniques, business tips, interpersonal relationship mechanics, and medical skills that will help you to stay organized and be successful and highly sought-after in our field.

In this book, I promise to give helpful techniques and pearls of wisdom that will aid you in your career path. We will talk about getting the best PA job for you, working with patients, doctors, and staff, as well as easy clinical practices and organization tips you can incorporate into your everyday work environment. I have many engaging and hard-learned lessons to share with you. You are welcome to learn from my mistakes and successes, or you can just have a cool book to display on your shelf. However, if you are ready for an encouraging, entertaining, and helpful journey, come along with me!

Warning: Side effects may include nausea, vomiting, diarrhea, lack of sleep, loss of appetite, headache, etc.

Chapter 1

Taking Purpose-Driven First Steps After Graduation

You don't have to be great to start,
but you have to start to be great.

—*Zig Ziglar*
Motivational speaker

Are We There Yet?

No one will tell you that it's not a huge accomplishment and undertaking to get into, go through, and graduate from PA school. No one could even call it a drive-by experience. At times, PA training can be difficult and grueling, but you have gotten through it like many others. Welcome to your career journey. Congratulations! You are in one of the most popular and highly growing professions there is. Like any other thing we do in life, there is still more to learn about being a PA and practicing medicine. So, in reality, you are there. You have arrived. What I'm trying to do, though, is to challenge you to be more than just 'there' in your career. Chose to be ever-present, ever-growing, and always purpose-driven!

What's Your Why?

Several years ago, one of my co-workers recommended the book, *Start With Why* by Simon Sinek. He told me that it changed his life and viewpoint of work. One day, I was on a long drive and decided to listen to the Audible version. It is an incredible book and has helped me immensely. It encourages you to find your why in everything you do: your home life, work-life, and within relationships.

Since junior high, I wanted to go into medicine to help people, and combine my love of medicine with doing something good for others. My why is knowing that I use my knowledge of medicine, science, compassion, and empathy to make someone else's life better than it was before they met me. After a leadership training course with Medtronic, I promised myself and those I've worked with in each situation. "Be Excellent. Care Greatly. Never Stop Learning."

With all the crazy of PA school, is there any chance you have forgotten your why? Why did you want to go? What was it about the career that got you excited? How passionate did you feel when you were interviewing? Do you still have that passion and that excitement about your profession?

I strongly encourage you to start every day with your why, your purpose, and your passion. Envision how it makes you feel to help, support, educate, and coordinate care for your patients that depend on you. Make a note of it and look at it often or write it down daily, so you don't forget why you do what you do. It will help you in your attitude, compassion, and determination for the day.

What's Your Why?
Have you forgotten your why in life?
Why did you want to go to PA school?
What about the PA career excites you?
What was your passion like when you were thinking of becoming a PA?
Do you still have that passion and excitement about your job?

Goal Digger

Have you set other goals since you first started your PA journey, aside from passing your tests and literally just getting through school? Speaking for myself, I pretty much dropped everything once I started. I stopped calling friends, I ignored my family, and working out was rare. I knew I needed to, but I became overwhelmed with learning everything I was taught—trying to keep up with coursework and clinical demands. I totally sucked at keeping everything together.

Three months before PA school started, I got married. Looking back, I can tell you that I did not start the marriage off well by being all-consumed with school. I did not make the important people in my life a priority. I failed to set daily goals. I did not remind myself of what I truly wanted to accomplish each day or how I wanted to feel at the end of each day. I simply made a few to-do lists, and started with the easy tasks, instead of tackling the most important and challenging things first when my brain had a better functioning capacity.

Hopefully, you were able to manage your time and relationships well, succeeding in setting goals inside and outside school. I want to encourage you to continue to set daily goals for yourself. That does not mean a to-do list. It entails both long-term and short-term goals, feelings, and attitudes you want to have towards your day and week, and long-term changes you want to work on.

Start your day focused on your why, where you want to go, and how grateful you are to be where you are, having all you have. You are incredible and have come a long way in your career aspirations.

If you are anything like me, it's difficult to remember what it is I wanted today to look like. I have to write it down or ask Siri to set a reminder for me, like calling the pest control guy. How are our goals any different? We have to keep our goals in front of us, as a reminder of the direction we want to go in.

How can we do this? Write them down. Start with a journal at home or work, and before you begin your day. Heck, keep one in both places, and if you forget in the morning, you can do it once you get to work. Make sure that your goals are important to you and inspire you.

So each day, jot down your why, write down three goals, and add something you are grateful for. This process will allow you to shape your perspective, your attitude and organize your day productively. And who doesn't need to start their day with gratitude? Being in a state of gratitude is life-changing.

I recently began keeping a journal in my bathroom, and while I'm getting ready, I write down what I am thankful for, along with a couple of goals. One recent entry reads: I am grateful for my kids, my husband, and my new front door (that took me forever to pick out and get installed). Under my goals section, you'll find: be present, work out, and don't eat anything fried today. This is seriously what's in it. It is not fancy or super detailed, and it was not even work-focused for the day, but it gives you an idea of my goofiness and maybe a place for you to start. Being intentional with goals has helped me set my mind up for success for the day.

If you have a patient list or to-do list at work where you enjoy crossing off your accomplishments for the day, you can even put some of your goals here if you don't have time to write them in a journal. The important thing is to keep your goals written down and in a place where you can see them on a consistent basis. Keep it on a Post-it® on your computer or bathroom mirror. Even if it's just one word to remind you, write it down! When you regularly write down your priorities, short-term and long-term goals and attitudes, this keeps them at the forefront of your mind, making you more likely to work on attaining them. What goal are you thinking about now?

Transitioning between school and your first PA job will be very exciting. Take the time to consider what you want in life, where you want to be, and who you want to be, making sure you start living the life you want. That is a perfect time to refocus.

Continue to strive for all that you desire.

Test Time

If you are just finishing up school or about to, then your PANCE test is right around the corner. I have never been as nervous as when I had to take that test. It didn't matter that our school had an excellent rate of first-time passing for the PANCE. I had never taken it, and I was a wreck. I spent too much time in the bathroom with pre-test diarrhea along with several other classmates. Have you been there too?

But, I'm here to tell you: You have what it takes. You will do well. You have made it this far, and you will succeed! See the chapter on certification for more insight.

Please know that if you do not pass the first time, you are not the only one to be in this situation. Many others have been in your shoes. Simply retake it as soon as you can, and focus on the areas where you did not perform well.

Pay Offs

Aren't you ready to make some money and—most importantly— start spending it? You have worked so hard and have sacrificed so much to get where you are today. You totally deserve to treat yourself well. Before you start spending that paycheck, though, consider doing a financial inventory. Are you in debt? When are your loans due? Who have you borrowed money from?

If you made it this far, you have no loans and are not in debt, keep rolling! That is fantastic!

If you are in the same boat, like so many others with loans galore, it may be time to start the loan repayment process sooner rather than later. Sit down, make a plan, and pay off those debts as soon as possible. Don't live with the debt hanging over your head, weighing on your mind and certainly, don't commit to a relationship or marriage without thoroughly discussing and developing a plan of attack for your debt. They may love and adore you, but I'm not so sure that will be the case for your student loans.

Fortunately, I did not have that much debt, as PA school was much cheaper when I went, but we were able to pay off the small loan within a few months of getting my first job. We did not buy a new car or a fancy house. Instead, we paid off the debt to get it out of the way as soon as possible.

I know of a doctor who was over $150,000 in debt when she got out of residency. She landed a job where she was making good money and decided to continue living on her resident budget until she had repaid her student loans. It only took her a few years, but she was super happy with this plan. I love this idea and have advised many people to do so. My son is about to go off to college without a scholarship and in a different state. He is interested in medical school. I'm sure that will mean loans and ramen noodles for him, but I keep stressing the importance of living a debt-free life as soon as you've got the chance.

I certainly don't have financial training, but I have made it a priority not to spend more money than I make, and never leave 401K cash on the table when a company is offering a matching program.

Seek financial wisdom from someone you trust. Find a financial planner to work with you. They can evaluate the size of the debt, the interest rates, and all that fancy stuff, and come up with an attainable plan of action. Even if you don't have a lot of money to invest upfront with them, they will see your potential and give you wise counsel as you are beginning to conquer your debt and start planning for your future retirement.

Do you owe anyone a debt of gratitude? Don't forget to thank those who have supported you through school. Also, you might want to thank them for not disowning you for forgetting birthdays, for forgiving you when you had to cancel plans at the last minute, and, for not being angry when you couldn't attend an important event. Can anyone relate?

We Don't Need No (More) Education; (Uhhhhh, Yes, you do)

PA programs are outstanding in teaching the fundamentals of medicine. I am so thankful for my experience. Even after all these years, I use specific techniques and skills I learned from my PA training every single day I practice. There is nothing like a solid foundation to build from. That said, PA school is a foundation for you to be an excellent provider at whatever practice you go into, be it general medicine or a subspecialty. After PA school, realize this is only the surface of your knowledge set, and you will need to continue on your pathway of learning.

You know as well as I do that there is new literature that comes out all the time. The practice of medicine today is so different from when I was in school in 1994. Medicine is ever-changing. In my career, I've had the opportunity to work with many specialists, and the ones who are excellent are the ones who continue to learn and read, putting into practice the most recent practice guidelines and performance measures. Don't just depend on your physicians to educate you. You should be reading the literature too. As PAs, we get multiple free journals sent to our house. I usually take a couple of minutes and read through my favorite, like derma dilemmas, and to take an ECG challenge. I guess that's only natural after spending nine years in cardiology. I like to know I've still got it even though I'm no longer looking at multiple ECGs every day. What are your favorite ones?

I see it as a challenge to eventually know as much—or more—as the physicians I work with. If they know I'm on top of my game and can easily discuss the recent literature and best practices with them, they can build more trust in me to care for our patients. You don't have to buy journals if you don't want to. Usually, your hospital has an online subscription, or your physician will have them in his or her office. You will be getting lots of free journals in the mail and will have so much access to articles online. You can also sign up for emails from journals and online magazines. They usually have brief articles that can be read in a minute or two.

As PAs, we have a lot of CME we are responsible for. One hundred hours every two years seems like a lot. However, there are CME earning and learning opportunities everywhere-online, in your area and fabulous locations across the country or even the world.

As I am writing this chapter, I am in a hotel room in Miami at a neurosurgery conference that starts tomorrow. If you are in a specialty, I highly recommend you go to conferences in your specialty. If you are unable to do so, you can visit the websites of some of the reputable schools. As I mentioned earlier, I worked in cardiology. I frequently would download CME from Texas Heart Institute and listen to their grand rounds and lectures for free. It was a great education and has benefited my patients and the way I practice medicine.

If you are in a medical center or hospital where they have grand rounds or teach fellows in your specialty, make it a priority, and go. Talk to your physician and let them know how helpful it will be. When I worked in gastroenterology, all of the physicians I worked with went to grand rounds each week, and they made it a requirement for me to go as well. I learned so much in such a short amount of time. The fellows you work with will probably have a required journal club. You may not have time to go to these, but try to get your hands on the articles they are discussing. They are often well-picked pertinent articles that are relatable for best practices.

Also, I encourage you to go to some of the pharmaceutical representatives' dinners or virtual presentations. They usually have excellent speakers, presenting fairly unbiased and engaging research as well as product information. It is up to you to keep up-to-date with recent guidelines and literature. These presentations can be quite helpful. And if they are in person, they are usually at very nice restaurants—education, wine and a meal, not such a bad deal.

Keeping Up With The Requirements

There are so many requirements to keep up with between the NCCPA and your state licensing board. However, the nice thing is that NCCPA reminds you of everything you need to be doing. When in doubt, just hop on their website and look up the information you need. All the dates and deadlines are there once you sign in. I usually keep track of them on my calendar as well.

The most time-consuming thing is logging your CME. Once you go to a conference, read an article, or go to grand rounds, immediately log your hours on NCCPA. At work, I keep a file with all of the category—one CME I have completed, in case of an audit.

I don't know a PA that has not scrambled at the end of the requirement cycle to make sure they have completed all the CME logging. It seems relatively common. Keep up with it the best you can, do a little every month. Some PAs listen to CME in the car, have apps on their phones, or listen to CME podcasts. This is a fast way to rake in the hours you need, especially since we don't get to go to multiple CME programs a year.

Keep up with state licensing as well. Go to your state's website and know the requirements. That should be easy, especially if there are fewer hours than NCCPA requires. And if you move states, make sure you have done your research before you do go!

My best recommendation for licensing and certification—Do not give it up. It takes so much time and effort to go back and recertify or get relicensed. Even if you change career paths, do your best to keep your certification current. Unfortunately, each state does not always send reminders. Register your home address instead of work because you want to ensure you get any reminders in a timely fashion.

Membership Has Its Privileges

There are many organizations that support PAs. There are local, states, national, and specialty PA organizations that are run by PAs just like you. These organizations are excellent resources to support you and the PA profession. They are a great way to meet other PAs and providers in your community and an excellent source for networking and learning how other practices in your field utilize PAs effectively. It might be a good idea to join these organizations while you are still a PA student because you will gain great insight on future job opportunities. You might also learn about the personality and nuances of the practice you are joining. It's a small world out there!

For most of my career, I have often been the only PA within my department or within my practice. To be honest, this can be quite isolating at times. It can be difficult to mesh well because it can seem like you don't really belong to the physician group or the nursing and ancillary staff group either. It is always a good to have another PA colleague to talk with and get ideas from. So make time to go to meetings that are close to you. If you don't have anything near you or in your field, start one! Ask the medical sales and device representatives to help you get the word out or even sponsor your event. Realize these guys are in and out of offices and hospitals and work with similar specialists all over town.

These organizations also have excellent CME opportunities and community outreach programs to get involved with.

As a PA, you have most likely been a leader all of your life. Don't let the opportunity pass you by to continue your leadership rolls by taking on an office within these organizations. It's also a great resume builder in case you need it for the future.

Once you leave PA school, your training as a PA will need to continue. I encourage you to continue to strive for excellence and persevere with your training and learning. Always seek to grow yourself. Strive to be the best in your field. Take ten to fifteen minutes at the beginning or end of each day to read a journal article or a book on your specialty. Find what you are not comfortable with and look for understanding in that area until you master it. Look for your weakest area first, then the second most vulnerable, and so on. You will be amazed at how much you can improve in such a short amount of time.

When I was going through my training, I never thought I would do cardiology or neurosurgery. I did not ever want to learn or interpret an ECG. I just prayed that the read out of the machine would say NORMAL SINUS RHYTHM. Now I've come to understand whatever ECG challenge is set before me, I see it as an opportunity to test my wicked ECG skills. I totally would never have guessed I would work in neurosurgery either. I look back and wonder who I am and who was that person making all the assumptions and limitations on my career? It's funny how we are sometimes thrust into situations and difficulties that always make us stronger and better individuals.

You are just beginning your journey as a PA. It's a big deal to finally get that C behind your name. It's the only time we are happy with this kind of letter grade. Right? Keep going. Keep dreaming. Keep reaching. By seeking out training and opportunities to improve yourself daily, your career will be off to an impressive future and you will be an expert in your field in no time.

Chapter 2

Taking Care of Yourself Before You Take Care of Others

Take care of yourself mentally, physically, and spiritually so that you can take care of the world.

—*Susan Love, MD*
American surgeon and prominent advocate of
preventive breast cancer research

If you are like so many other caregivers, taking care of a patient is the easy part, while ignoring yourself is even easier. Ignoring myself started early for me and got progressively worse when I went to PA school. You know how it is; PA school is really busy, really stressful and completely overwhelming.

Did I say overwhelming? I gained at least fifteen pounds! I did not make healthy eating choices, I was not exercising, and I completely neglected myself emotionally. I scheduled events and met up with friends, but I was not always present in the conversation. I think all I could focus on was the unhealthy balance of getting through school and learning all that I could. Hello! They are squishing four years of medical school, a year of internship, and residency into PA training. It is so much to take in. Getting through school was my only thought and priority! Then I got out of PA school, had two children, and the focus shifted to figuring out how to parent, work, clean, shop, and keep everything from being sticky and free of goldfish crumbles. I just did not think there was enough time to fit the things in that I needed to do for myself.

One day, as I was talking with one of my cardiology patients, advising him about weight loss, exercise, and taking care of himself, I felt as though he was giving me the once over. I was wondering why in the world he was looking at me like this and then I noticed he was looking at all of me. ALL OF ME—all of my overweight and all-around unhealthy self. That was undoubtedly an Oprah Aha moment. How in the world was anyone going to listen to me and take me seriously if I did not follow my advice that showed the positive results of exercising and eating well? Don't you think our patients would be more motivated if we followed our own advice? I mean, who are we to tell our patients what to do when we don't even stick to our most basic instructions? And that guy was just witnessing the external junk in my trunk. He had no idea of the disaster that lay underneath the surface.

I was a hot mess inside and out!

Why do we not take care of ourselves? Every time you fly, the flight attendant always tells you to put your oxygen mask on first before you assist anyone else. You know you can't take care of others unless you take care of yourself.

I cannot stress it enough: you can't take care of others unless you take care of yourself!

You should let this sink in. If you are a PA, you are a caregiver at work and in your personal life. You probably think about every-one in your life and do everything for everyone else and do very little for yourself, because really after you've done everything for everyone else, is there even anything left over for you? Think about this.....What is the last thing you did for yourself? Yes, you and no one else? The next question is do you even know what to do for yourself that you enjoy? Are these difficult questions for you to answer? If so, you know I am talking to you!

You need to take care of yourself in all aspects of your life. Get yourself together so you can help others help themselves. Your physical, emotional, and spiritual health is vital, and if no one has told you recently, you are worthy of doing good things for yourself!

Physically—just do it!

If you are overweight from poor habits and harping on your patients to lose weight, make good eating choices and exercise, I'm sure they are looking at you like you are crazy too. I am not here to body shame or to condemn you in any way at all. I am here to encourage you to make healthier choices. Most of us probably don't want to hire an out of shape personal trainer, so why would our patients want to take advice from us when we don't follow it ourselves? I used to think the ugliest thoughts about my high school basketball coach and his out-of-shape self, having us run lines on the basketball court. Acting like he just did twenty of them before we got there, so it should be easy for us. We all want to be coached by someone walking the walk.

The truth is, we all make judgments on the way people take care of their bodies. That's what we do as PAs; we assess what is going on with our patients and help them address it. If we can change them from the inside, it will eventually show up on the outside. We are in the business of judging others, objectively as possible, and then advising on how to come up with a plan to make them happier and healthier. In a way, we think that what we suggest should be easy for our patients to follow and get great results if they would just stick to our advice!

Exercise is just like that. Just do it! Take the time. Make yourself a priority and get moving at least thirty consecutive minutes a day. I truly believe that exercise is one of the best medicines. It makes you feel better, and when you feel better, you do better. You don't need to look like a supermodel or that you just stepped out of a fabulous Instagram shoot. Just knowing that you are taking care of yourself and having the confidence from that, that is enough. I know I am less irritable when I work out, and I love the sense of knowing that I am making long-term positive changes for my health.

These days, there are many different programs for all kinds of people. I used to get so motivated when I saw infomercials on working out! I would sit there watching Beachbody and Tony Horton's P90X, P90X3, and loved their clients' transformations. Now we are pretty much commercial-free, but there are folks out there with specific workouts and quick workouts on Amazon and Netflix and just about every other place that you can stream anywhere and anytime. Whether you work out at a gym or home, whether you work out in the morning (bless your heart) or at night, find something that works for you and get to it!

Keep trying new things until you find what works for you and gets you energized. Just the other day, I told my son that it is called a work out for a reason. There is work in a workout! It's not easy. But who doesn't feel better getting a good exercise in and getting some of that daily stress out? I find that if I don't work out as soon as I get home, I will not do it. Even in my fancy workout leggings, if my butt hits the couch, I'll end up moving from one end of the couch to the other to avoid pressure ulcers. Find your best time, and stick with it.

Diners, Drive-Ins, and Dives

The English writer Virginia Woolf said, "One cannot think well, love well, sleep well if one has not dined well." I love this quote, and it's so true. What we eat is the foundation of how we feel. Several years ago, one of the gastroenterologists I worked with told me about the book, *The Mind-Gut Connection* by Emeran Mayer. It is a fantastic and easy read and talks about food, how we perceive it, and the importance of our choices. I implemented some of the thoughts into both my son and my diet, and I have noticed a positive difference. When he was dealing with depression, I was somewhat desperate, trying to change anything I could to help him. I am confident that the positive change in diet was instrumental in him getting on the road to feeling better. And I felt better too.

I might be writing this to you, but in truth, I am writing this to remind myself as well. This is one of the biggest struggles I have up to this day. I love junk food and just about anything bad for me. Constantly, I seem to crave chili cheese Fritos and frozen custard with key lime pie. Not at the same time, but possibly in the same day. I love to eat and eat a lot. But, I am telling you, once you start on a consistent journey of eating more healthy options, you will find that you will feel so much better and have much more energy. This is a relatively new concept for me as I have gone back and forth with dieting for so long. Over the last years, if I lapse into my poor diet, there's a noticeable change in my mood, body, and skin.

There will be times when you eat everything in sight or want to, but just do the best you can daily. And if you mess up, don't beat yourself up. Just get back on track the next day. Make a few changes here and there and work on getting rid of the junk in your diet. This will look different for all people.

I try to work on eating healthy six days a week, and then, on one day on the weekend, I usually eat what I want to for the most part. Please don't ask my husband if I follow this, he might say otherwise, but I *do* try. Have you seen Dwayne 'The Rock'

Johnson and what he eats? I follow him on Instagram, so I know his cheat day is Sunday. His meals vary from a heaping platter of sushi to a fiesta of French toast that is basically two loaves of bread. Those are crazy meals, but you can't deprive yourself all the time. Simply find a solution that works well for you with family and career.

If you have a large office, there is always a reason to celebrate someone's birthday, wedding, divorce, or baby shower. There will always be cakes, cookies, and treats to indulge in. And then there are the sales reps who bring in some of the most delicious fattening foods from the best bakeries. Consider celebrating and enjoying the occasion without regularly partaking in the sweets. If reps bring food into the office, have them bring in healthy options as well. Who cares if your staff isn't too crazy about it? It will set a good example for them.

Since I have been in the industry and have been in two states worth of GI offices, I will tell you that I have noticed that there is a big—and I mean *big*—difference in the offices who have reps in every day for several meals and the ones that don't. I realize that you are stressed and overworked. It easy to reward yourself with the special treats lying around, but I am urging you to try and avoid that mindset. Reward yourself with good things. And really, are those treats going to make you feel better forty-five minutes after you eat them?

Being healthy is a choice, a daily choice, a meal-by-meal choice. Keep making the right decisions, and they will incrementally add up. If you want to meet with a rep, but—like me—you are easily distracted by unhealthy choices, consider walking with them around your medical complex. That way, you learn something, socialize, and get a break from your day to help you refocus on your next patients and tasks.

I Wanna Thank Me

My friend, you deserve some time and relaxation and soul service! You need to allow yourself some down-time, alone time, me time, or whatever you call it, or it calls to you. How do you relax, rejuvenate, and reenergize? Do you even know? I think this can be a difficult question for so many of us, but it deserves some contemplation and then lots of attention.

I think I am still figuring this out. There are so many time stealers where I think I am relaxing, but in reality, after I am done with them, I don't feel better. Sometimes, I watch movies or TV series with my kids, and I just don't feel that great afterward. They stress me out. And then I realize I am not entertained or even intrigued. I have not learned anything, and I just feel icky inside even though I plopped down on the couch to relax and watch them. Does that happen to you? Do you think you are relaxing with social media or television time and realize that it does absolutely nothing for you? Maybe not, but work on finding what *speaks* to you and gives you rest.

With all the apps out there for just about everything, have you tried any that help you meditate? I love some of the five to ten-minute ones that are guided and take you through several steps like focusing on being grateful, mindful, or kind toward others. I have downloaded meditations from Audible and from various apps like *Breathe* or *Calm*. I like to lie down on my floor in my room and meditate after I exercise. I find it very relaxing and sometimes reenergizing after a tough workout. There are also meditations for sleep that are fantastic and super helpful. By centering on someone's voice, your mind does not wander as much, and you get rid of the stress from the day and keep tomorrow's worries in tomorrow.

Resting and getting a good night's sleep is good for you. You already know it refuels you and gives you strength for the next day. With all the options we have to record and watch shows at a later time, could you save time by watching shows at an appropriate time for you without the commercials? And social media are we ridiculous? Do you really care about what your college roommate's best friend made for dinner or how your daughter's friend's hair looked after her fancy blow out in Chicago? The posts and tweets will be there tomorrow. When it is late, and you are exhausted, put your phone away and get some rest.

I truly believe—and I'm still trying to apply this in my own life—that if we treat ourselves right and make the best of our prime hours of the day, we will not allow ourselves unhealthy me-time with television and social media at night. Intentionally plan to give yourself quality time to reflect and regroup.

Mind Over Matter

Tony Robbins is one of my absolute favorite motivational speakers and life coaches. He is remarkable, serving so many of the underserved. He has a saying that has changed my life. "Trade your expectation for appreciation and the world changes instantly." Your emotional well-being is as important as any other aspect of your life. According to self-growth.com, emotional well-being is not the absence of emotions, but your ability to understand the value of your feelings and use them to move your life in positive directions.

While lying in bed at night, do you ever replay your day? Do you say to yourself, "I should have said this or done that?" If you're like me, you can't easily let go of specific events of the day. For example, you might still be upset about flinging your son's iPod across the room because he never checked his pockets before bringing the laundry down. That was a long time ago—hence the iPod—but you know what I mean. Quite often, I have replayed in mind interactions with patients and colleagues, regretting some of the things I said, despite knowing I'll never have that conversation again. In many instances, I repeat conversations out loud in the kitchen while cooking dinner, and when my kids ask me who I am talking to. I admit, I am rephrasing things or apologizing because I might have stuck my foot in my mouth, asking a patient's wife to wait for her son outside. Can we all just agree that we need to forgive ourselves and not replay things in our head? Give yourself a break. Evaluate what you will do better next time, forgive yourself, and let it go.

Spiritually speaking, I am a Christian, and I believe in God and Jesus. Reading the bible, studying its lessons, and embracing the hope it offers, has been life-changing for me. No matter what your religion is, take time to focus on your inner peace, strength, meaning, and contribution. Your spiritual well-being will most likely look different than anyone else's. Spirituality is deeply personal and is vital to ensure a consistent source of meaning, peace, hope, and how we confront the daily trials in our life. Seek out different avenues and find what speaks to you and what can help you daily. Pursue it regularly.

I follow several inspirational and positive people and organizations on Instagram. Seeing a motivational quote in the morning puts me in the right mindset for beginning my day.

Continue to build your own support system. Make time for friends that minister to you and build you up, and focus on being a friend as well. When I was going through my divorce in 2007, I started going to a counselor, and I still go from time to time. For me, seeing a therapist has helped me professionally and personally by giving me an objective viewpoint on some very stressful situations that not all of my friends or family could relate to. We all need someone to talk to about our stressors. Talk to someone even if you have to pay for it. At least you know they will be present and engaged with what you are saying. I promise it will be worth every dime you spend! Remember, you are worth it.

You have to take time to figure out what motivates, encourages you, and feeds your soul. Ask yourself what gives you energy, or as Marie Kondo asks, "What sparks joy?" Is it a self-help book, a motivational podcast, a vacation out in nature, a walk with your loved one, or a friend that sparks joy for you? We all know that sometimes our patients' situations can suck the life out of us, but it's up to us to not to allow that to happen, by keeping our emotional well-being strong and nurtured.

Are you rolling over your unused vacation every year? It is time to start using it! Maybe save a couple of days in case of an emergency. But really, take some time for you even if it is a staycation. I have always struggled to take a vacation because I don't always plan it out, and by the time I do want to take it, someone else has requested that same period. I know it is a pain in the butt, but try to schedule your vacation time early on in the year, especially if you have to work around your coworkers. You deserve time off to focus on you and your family.

My youngest and I like to quote Tom and Donna from the series Parks and Recreation, "Treat yo self." In the show, they make it a point of going out on occasion and treat themselves with massages, fancy clothes, a night out, or whatever else strikes their fancy. You need to do that too. You work hard and make good money. Take some of that and do nice things that are meaningful to you. There's a pretty good chance you will find me at my local TJ Maxx, Nordstrom Rack, or the Wine Store. Just sayin'.

Choosing to take care of yourself is essential for you, your family, and your patients. Address all aspects of your life and become the best possible version of you so that you can contribute fully. Small simple positive choices are all it takes. You deserve your best.

Chapter 3

Getting the PA Job You Want

People don't leave bad jobs, they leave bad bosses.
—LinkedIn

◆ ◆ ◆

Train people well enough so they can leave,
treat them well enough so they don't want to.
—Richard Branson

Y ou are in one of the hottest careers on the market, and you deserve the best job for you. I sometimes think when we get out of PA school; we are just looking for a job to start paying our student loans, and get rid of the clunker of a car that we have been driving since high school. I am telling you, and all your PA mentors will agree: Don't settle on anything that doesn't work for you. You are too good for that, and you have worked way too hard to take a job that you know you are not going to like. Take your time and be wise about your choices. Make a choice based on what you want to do. I know that is not so easy in small towns where options might be limited, but do your research and know that you are interviewing them as much as—if not more—than they are interviewing you. It seems that there are way more PA jobs than there are PAs.

First, make a list of all the things you are looking for in a job and what you are willing to accept.

Questions to ask when looking for a PA Position
How do I envision myself in this career?
Which days of the week do I want to work?
What type of hours do I want to work on?
Do I want to be on call?
Do I want to work at weekends?
What type of practice do I picture myself in?
Do I want to work only in outpatient?
Do I want to be in a surgical setting?
Do I want inpatient and outpatient?
Does this practice have loan repayment opportunities?
What is the salary?
Do I want a job with a salary and commission?
What type of environment do I want?
Do I want hospital, clinic, rural, large, or small practice?
What am I willing to give up to get the ideal job I want?
What do I want long term? Does the job I want now fit into that plan and give me that opportunity in the future?

Looking For Jobs in All the Right Places

There are many ways to go about looking for a job in our profession and there are a ton of PA jobs out there. Here are some thoughts on how to go about looking for a job.

Academic Access

If you are a new or soon-to-be graduate, your school most likely has a source for you to look for job opportunities. This can be extremely helpful. Also, if there is a listing at your school, then most likely, those opportunities are from practices and physicians who are willing to train and work with new graduates, which is fantastic. As a new graduate, it is essential to work with a physician or group of physicians who are willing to train you.

As you are going through your clinical rotations, keep in mind that this might be an opportunity to secure a position with the practice or hospital you are working with. Several of my PA friends received job offers from the practices they worked while they were still students. It was perfect. The practice had an idea of how the student was going to be as a full-time employee, and the student had an idea of how well they could work with the practice. You might consider trying to get some of your clinical rotations in a location, and a practice you are interested in joining. You receive top-notch training, and the practice gets a trial-run to see if you are a good fit. It's a win-win situation!

Every rotation you are on is a job interview and a potential good or bad reference in the making. A PA once told me that an administrator with the hospital she works with called about a student she worked with during one of the student's clinical rotations. The administrator wanted a reference, but unfortunately, the student hadn't made a good impression on the PA for many reasons. He wasn't on time and didn't seem interested in learning. Needless to say, the new PA did not get the job. So, I'm just saying, make every interaction you have on your rotations count.

Local and State Associations and AAPA

There are great listings for jobs within your local, state, and national associations. And yes, it is worth the price of joining to get access to job listings if not available without a membership. In any case, you should join for all kinds of other benefits we talk about in other areas of the book, but let's focus on getting a job right now. The specialty organizations will be able to help you focus on getting that particular position you are looking for. If there are no job listings on their sites, you can also research who the officers of the organization are by looking through the website. Definitely reach out to them and see if they can help you.

Special Agents

Working with a recruiter can be extremely helpful in finding the perfect job. Recruiters are like having an agent. If Patrick Mahomes has an agent, why shouldn't you? Recruiters find the best qualities in you and will represent your best attributes and what you have to offer to the hospital or practice. They have a vested interest in helping you get the job you want. When they seek you out via LinkedIn or just call you up randomly (how they get our numbers, I have no idea), they are usually looking for a specific candidate with experience for the positions they are trying to fill.

Realize that they get paid by the practice that is looking for the PA, so unlike the athletes who pay their agents, you will not need to spend any money. In many instances, I have gotten a call out of the blue by recruiters. I always call back and find out what they are looking for because it's best to keep an open mind. You never know, they may have the position you have been looking for with the ideal group and more money. It never hurts to talk with them and review your options. Sometimes you can use a job offer to renegotiate with your current practice. Regardless, it is good practice to be respectful and call them back, whether you are interested in the opportunity or not. You just might need them in the future. If you are relocating, they might have national connections and can represent you.

Search Engine Optimization

There are all kinds of online sources available to find jobs. Indeed, LinkedIn, and so many greater job sites are right at your fingertips. If you are interested in working for a certain hospital system, go to their specific site and check out their opportunities as well. Sometimes they do not advertise as much.

Make sure that if you apply for a position online, you call or email the contact person to introduce yourself, ensure that they received your information, and ask if they need any clarifications from you. That will start a good rapport, show your initiative, and make you stand out as opposed to other candidates who just email their information randomly without proper follow up. Follow-up is super important no matter what stage in the job search you are in.

Phone A Friend

If you know a PA in a specialty that you are interested in, make sure you use them as a valuable resource and recommendation. They may have some insight on whom to contact or call, as well as specific opportunities with their practice or others they are aware of. Also, they might advise you on whom not to work for. Being employed in some practices or hospitals might not be a good idea, considering their reputation for poor patient care or disreputable physicians and specialties. Unfortunately, some practices are well-known for how poorly they treat their PAs and staff. Do your research, call around, and connect with other PAs on social media to help you find the best opportunity. Even if the practice you are interviewing with hasn't had a PA before, you can look into its reputation and physicians' before joining. Be creative, do your homework. It will be worth it.

Uncle Sam Wants You

The Veteran's Administration (VA) is the largest employer of PAs in the nation. Working for the government, either as a civilian or service member, should be a consideration for you. Within government service, there are options to work for the federal prison system, The Indian Health Service, the VA, and the armed services.

There are excellent benefits to working in federal service. When you work for the government, you are not only providing for your own family but for the men and women who have served and protected the United States of America. As a PA who worked for the VA for over 12 years, it was an honor to serve our veterans. Unlike federal service, many small practices and some hospitals do not offer retirement packages, healthcare packages, and vacation benefits. As a PA for the VA, I earned 26 days of vacation a year, 13 days of sick leave, and 10 paid holidays. The VA has also come into this century in their pay scales for PAs as well. They are definitely competing for great PAs to come work for them. They match 401k contributions up to 5%. I am here to tell you that a 5% match on 401K is tough to find in the healthcare setting. A couple of the companies I have worked for in the industry can't even compare to that. Remember, you have to start saving early for retirement. You missed a pivotal contribution time while you were attending school.

If you want to work on student loan repayment and get it done fast, working for the government might be a good option for you. Talk to the government recruiter to find out more and if the position you are considering would qualify for loan repayment.

Some PAs work a regular job and then join the reserves as a way to get an extra income. And by extra, it is nothing to sneeze at. The military usually has excellent sign-on bonuses and significant benefits, some including loan repayment plan whether you join the reserves or go in as a full-time officer. If you are interested in any of these, go to usajobs.gov (login. gov), or for specific military service, you can look online or go to your local recruiter office.

Nurse Practitioner Positions

When I first moved to Kansas City in 2004, I contacted a recruiter I found online, and she sent my resume to a practice that was looking for an NP. I ended up working for their practice for a year and a half. I was the only PA working with three nurse practitioners and twelve cardiologists.

If you are interested in a specific job and it is listed as a nurse practitioner position, I would recommend applying for it. What do you have to lose? In my opinion, it has taken a while for my state to become more PA-friendly, and I thought I had few options. So, I thought I would see if they would hire and work with a PA instead of an NP. See it as an opportunity to educate the interviewer as to what physician assistants can do and how we provide the most excellent service for our patients.

Some jobs are posted as Advanced Practice Provider (APP) positions as well and are open to both NP and PAs. Don't forget to use APP in your search in addition to PA searches when you are looking online.

Social Butterfly

Now that you have applied to that wonderful job you have found, you might want to have a couple of things taken care of before your prospective employee, even looks at your resume or application. First and foremost, you should probably take a look at your social media and determine if anything needs to be deleted. Are there some inappropriate pictures of you online, or is there a chance you have been tagged in some? You might just want to sort through your tweets, posts, places tagged, and TikTok dances or rants you might have forgotten all about. Always be who you are. But if you do feel uncomfortable with a future employer looking at those items, simply delete what you can.

With all of the COVID 19 chaos, I lost my job and was looking for another one. Some of the institutions and organizations asked my URL for Facebook, Twitter, and LinkedIn. I am not super exciting, but if they like looking at my children and me at Planet Comicon or photos of my 2019 nuptials and a 2015 tweet about the Kansas City Royals winning the World Series, then by all means, go for it. I am not saying I have not done anything I wouldn't want to be posted all over the place. I just haven't shared those potentially embarrassing events… yet.

Trust me; employers will look at your social media pages. It is likely part of the HR protocol for evaluating candidates. I have no idea, but since they are asking for the info on some applications now, just take this into consideration. I guess this is one of the reasons why my child has four different Instagram accounts with entirely off-the-wall usernames?

I Want To Be A Part Of It

My dear friend Kim, who has been in sales for many years, has taught me a precious lesson in getting what you want. She always—and I mean always—says, "Rachel, if you don't ask, the answer is always no." If you know of a physician, practice, or hospital you want to work for, don't hesitate to call the practice administrator or the physician/physicians to express your interest. Seek them out at conferences, in the hospital, or online. It shows initiative and that you are specifically interested in working for them.

Not every PA job is advertised. Some practices and physicians always considered having a PA, but have not taken the initiative to look for one. They can be so lazy sometimes. Some of these offices just don't know how beneficial a PA can be to their practice. So get yourself out there and tell them what a great asset you will be to their practice. You could even put together a business proposal on the benefits of hiring a PA and make it specific to their practice. They don't know what they don't know.

It's worth a try. If they don't want you, it is totally their loss! Move on to your next target and conquer.

Using Your Reputation

Having an excellent reputation will get you all kinds of job offers. Several of the job offers I have received have been from physicians that I have worked with in some capacity. While in cardiology, I regularly worked with primary care providers and surgeons. We all worked together to coordinate care for our mutual patients. They developed a respect for the care their patients received from me. I would have them tell me frequently that I could come and work with them any day.

Actually, this is how I ended up in neurosurgery. The neurosurgeons approached me several times while I was in cardiology, asking if I would come to work with them. Then, one day when they caught me in the hallway, said they would work with my schedule, teach me new skills, and I would be part of their close-knit operation. I think I kept saying no to them because I was afraid of being in neurosurgery and did not know if I had what it took. I knew it would be a great challenge for me, but to be completely honest, I wanted to work for them. They all had a great reputation as excellent physicians and surgeons, and they are known for being kind to their staff. It was a great decision. They totally worked with my schedule and I loved being part of their team.

When you develop a good rapport with the physicians and providers you work with on a regular basis, and having patients talk favorably about you, I promise that your reputation will precede you. Every interaction is a possibility of a job in the future. You never know when your doctor is going to drop dead in Fiji while on vacation like one of mine did, leaving you to look for your next gig. Seriously, I had to clean out his office, and I learned all kinds of interesting things about him. All I'm saying is to be kind, build a good rapport with those you work with, and always consider new opportunities when they present themselves.

Speaking of building rapport and networking, use the student relationships you have as leverage for your first or next PA position. When I went through training at Baylor College of Medicine, we had several classes with medical students, such as anatomy and pharmacology. We also had our rotations with them all over town. We were all doing the same job as students. The medical students see how hard PA students work and know PAs usually have more classes than they do because PA programs seriously compress medical school into a short amount of time. They know how extensive your training has been because you were right there beside them all along. These students will be the hiring doctors one day. They know your value and respect your training.

I would encourage you to make friends with the med students. You might end up working for them, or they might be working for your practice one day. Regardless, strategic networking can be the key to finding the right position.

Know Your Numbers

I strongly encourage you to do your research before accepting any position. When you settle for less than you are worth, you do yourself and our profession a great disservice. You have worked way too hard to settle for less than you are worth. Realize that whoever you are working for is in business to make money, and they will try to acquire you for the least amount possible. You are in business to enjoy your career and family and get paid the most money possible for the quality work you bring to your position.

Do your homework. Every year we fill out a census for AAPA on salaries, hours worked, bonuses, etc. (this is a good time for me to encourage you to fill this out every year. It is beneficial for our profession, especially in negotiating salaries.) This information is an excellent leveraging tool and is available at AAPA.org. In essence, it breaks down information on average wages for PAs, among new graduates, specialties, states, etc. and contains invaluable information. I have used it several times as an objective tool to negotiate a reasonable salary.

If you are an above-average PA, do not settle on a below-average salary. It is up to you to know your worth. Don't be afraid to counter offer. I had the privilege of auditing an MBA level course in negotiations at Northwestern University several years ago. I learned many things in this course, and one of them is to 'anchor high.' If you are asked what your expectant salary is, be fair, but also ask for more than what you would ultimately settle for.

This anchoring will set expectations and be a signal to them that they will not be giving the bargain basement PA salary that they would like to. If they don't pay you what you are worth, that's more money in their pockets. If you ask for a little more and they come back and say they can't do it, they will at least know what your expectations are. They need to realize what you will be bringing to their practice or hospital and pay you accordingly. If you have a back-up offer, use it to negotiate an appropriate salary for yourself and those who follow in your footsteps. I know it can be scary to do this, and it is entirely uncomfortable. They are fully aware of this, and sometimes they offer a lot less because of that. They are counting on the fact that you might want to avoid having a conversation to negotiate a decent salary. Chin up. Stand up for yourself and your skills. You can do it!

Many negotiation aspects are far beyond the topics of this book, but some of the critical elements are below:

Everything is negotiable…even if you think it isn't.

Know what is most important to you and your employer. It may be they only have $90,000 in their budget and your expectant salary is $104, 000. If they can't work out of their 90k, then negotiate more vacation, bonuses, fewer hours, or a combination. You can accept that job, but ask every Friday afternoon off to compensate for what you lack in salary. If you can't figure out what's important to them, just ask.

Before you go for broke, consider your BATNA (Best Alternative to a Negotiated Agreement). If you have a better job offer, it might be worth playing a little at the negotiating table. What do you have to lose? Especially if you already have something lined up that you are happy with. If a recruiter is calling you to see if you will take a job across town, why not negotiate or put a request out there for them? Ask yourself what it would take to accept this position over the other position and then ask for it. You truly have nothing to lose if you already have a good option.

However, if there is no other job offer for you within months or miles, you will have to be a little more delicate with your negotiating skills. I'm not saying to go in and be ruthless at all. Always be professional, but don't be afraid to ask for what you want. And never ever burn your bridges.

First Impressions

Since you've made it to PA school, your interviewing skills are already excellent. I thought I would go over some essential items that are a little more PA-specific you might want to consider.

First of all, dress for success! You should be dressed at the level of who is interviewing you or better. I would suggest a nice professional suit that is new and fashionable and shoes that are not scuffed or old. Do not wear tight clothing, ladies. You may look fantastic in that skintight animal-print dress, but do you want to deal with a boss that hired you because of your sexy dress? Please, please, please, dress appropriately. And if, for some reason, someone calls and wants to interview you on the same day, and you are in scrubs or your least favorite outfit, address your clothing very briefly when you walk in the door. I have done several same-day job interviews while wearing scrubs.

Have fresh breath as well. Appearance and fresh breath are crucial not only to an interview but to your everyday relationships! Unless we are still in this COVID phase of mask wearing, then I guess this part really doesn't matter. I'm so goofy and always afraid my patients will think my breath is bad that I sometimes hold my breath as I am examining them. Then I get all out of breath… It's a ridiculous behavior but who wants Diet Coke and Chili Cheese Frito breath wafted in their direction? Have you ever had a healthcare provider with bad breath?

You should be at least fifteen minutes early for your interview. I usually plan for the worst-traffic scenario. If I'm early, I sit in the parking lot or garage and make a list of all my questions I want to ask. I also review any research I may have done about that practice or hospital. You can also evaluate how you plan to get up to speed with practice guidelines for the disease states you will be treating. If you are doing an online interview via Zoom or some app, join the meeting at the exact time or one to two minutes before. Sometimes there can be other candidates that are interviewing, and times may overlap.

Have a portfolio with at least several copies of your resume available for review and printed on quality paper. Do not use regular paper. Invest in some from Office Depot or even send it to them. They can print it off on quality paper faster than if you went up to buy it, brought it home, and got your printer to work to find out you are out of ink. It's happened. Trust me! Many times I have been in interviews where the physicians have not even reviewed my resume beforehand, and no one bothered to make copies for them. You will be thankful you have many on hand. Sometimes you may even interview with more people than you expected.

Have a firm handshake and make direct eye contact frequently.

Have a list of questions available that you want to ask them. Make sure to ask key questions that will be important in your decision-making process. Here are a few points that I think will help with your job choices.

Questions to ask during a PA interview
Tell me about your practice
Tell me about the payor mix (Medicare, Medicaid, Private, Self-Pay)
What are some of the biggest challenges you face in your practice?
How do you see my skill set fitting in, and where can I take on additional roles to help?
What is the best way to approach you when I have questions, and the patient is in the office?
What are some things I can be doing now to prepare for this job before I join?
What kind of supervision will be provided?
What does a typical week look like in the practice?
What are the hours like?
How often is call?
For call, is it at home or at the hospital?
With whom will I be on call?
Is call part of the salary, or is it extra? (You may want to save specific money questions for after the job has been offered)
How approachable are the physicians when asked questions, and how rapid is the response time?
How many locations/satellite offices will I be covering?

These are just a few points for you to consider as you prepare for your interview. Add to the list here, or write down some questions in your portfolio before walking in. If you will be working for more than one physician, ask them some of the same questions and see if their answers match. You can consider finding a way to ask the other staff members, PAs or NPs as well.

Personally, I would ask about coverage and if you have to work your vacation around the other providers. Nothing stinks as much as needing a certain day or week off and someone else decided to take off every other Friday for the summer and you both can't be off at the same time. Of course they put their request in in January ahead of yours so theirs is approved. So now you have to figure out how to work your custody schedule with your kid's dad and the Friday vacation day hog. They are out there!

If you have recently graduated, I would recommend choosing a job where the physician is readily available and easily accessible. This will help in boosting your confidence and decision-making capabilities. If you have the impression that immediately after PA school, you are ready to practice in a rural capacity or with limited supervision, I don't care who you are, you are wrong!

If you are entering a new specialty or new position or are a new grad, you will need to ask what their approach will be for your training.

You will want to have some thoughtful questions about their business, strategy, and goals to help you stand out above the others. You want to let them know you will be there for the long term, that you want to be successful, and help their practice while they are running a business and taking care of patients. You also want them to know you can be valuable to them in other areas as well. Make yourself indispensable. Let them know that you get the big picture, and you are willing to be a part of the more significant cause.

Sometimes you might be asked a two or three-part question, and you may feel like you got sidetracked by answering just one. If something like that happens, simply ask, "Does that answer your question?" Whoever is interviewing you, they will redirect you. Or just say that you forgot the second or third part of the question. Asking if they got what they needed or need further clarification will give them another opportunity if you didn't quite get everything the first time. I can't tell you how many times I've had to ask interviewers to repeat the question. I've learned to jot a note down to remind myself of the question to keep me on track.

Taking notes during the interview is a must. It shows you're both interested and serious about the position. Write down their expectations, hours, responsibilities, questions, or concerns that come up during your interview. Remember, you are interviewing them as much as they are interviewing you. You will spend a lot of time at work, so make sure they are a good fit. I want to make sure my work-family is more functional than my dysfunctional extended family.

Remember, you get to choose your work family!

After interviewing, always send a thank-you note or email that mentions something personal about your interview. It's important to remind them of anything you formed a bond or found common ground over. Even if it's that you enjoyed learning about their passion for collecting taxidermied animals, send something fun, yet professional. This will ensure they will remember you and hopefully remind them they need to get that offer out to you before you choose a different job.

Who's Your Daddy?

Okay, this one may seem a little strange, but it is essential to know who your boss is. Who has the hiring power and firing power? Since I worked in the VA system, the doctors I worked with were my bosses, but could not necessarily fire me. I worked for several VAs for over 12 years and can't tell you who I directly reported to. In one of the private practices I worked for, I never knew if I worked for the office manager who was always in everyone's business or for the two doctors that interviewed me and who I worked with on a daily basis.

Simply ask who you will be reporting to and who will be doing reviews. Sometimes it's glaringly obvious, but with large organizations, it can be confusing. Just the other day, a PA friend called me and told me their administration informed them they were getting a new physician added to their practice. The other physicians did not even interview the doctor. As they later found out, the latest addition is married to a doctor, the hospital needed in another specialty. They hired two doctors to get the one they needed, and no one had a say in any of it. My friend told me that it was at that point, she understood that she didn't work for any of the doctors in her office.

It is important to know who you are working for. Network to find out about the practice and the personality of the physicians and staff you will be working with. You certainly don't need to know everything, but do some digging in case there is any pending litigation against the practice or physicians. Am I just paranoid? I don't know, but I can tell you that I don't want to work with someone who is frequently named in lawsuits. Orange is definitely not my new black.

Shake Your Moneymaker

Let's get down to more PA specifics. My friend, please realize that you are the prize! You are going to be the one that makes their practice run smoothly. You are going to be the front line of their practice. You have the training and are ready to make a difference for them! They will be lucky to have you. They may have the hiring decisions and the money, but you are the one that will be billing and bringing their practice more money. Be choosy! You need a job that is a good fit for you, your family, and the opportunities you want to pursue in the future.

You need to sell yourself with confidence. It can be a bit difficult to sell yourself, but you need to let them know you and the value you bring. Know your facts and represent yourself and your skills well. As a PA, you are a moneymaker because you bring wealth to the practice. You will do infinitely more than earning your keep. When I first worked in gastroenterology and performed about 50 flexible sigmoidoscopies a week, and saw 30–40 clinic patients a week, they were billing out a lot of money for my services and they were paying me a very poor salary. When I sat down and figured out the numbers and addressed my productivity with my physicians, they offered me a raise.

Calculate what you are billing out per week or month in your current position, so you can pass this information to the people you are interviewing with. If you know your numbers and what you are capable of, it will show them how profitable and productive you can be for their practice. If you are not aware of what you are currently billing, go to your medical coder within your office or organization and figure it out. Make friends with these folks. The billing and coding information is beneficial for negotiating salaries and selling yourself.

If other PAs or NPs are working for the practice or hospital, do not accept a position without speaking with at least one of them. They will be an important deciding factor for you to determine whether you are interested in working for a physician or practice. You can get a good feel for the practice environment after speaking with them. Ask questions you might not feel comfortable voicing to the physicians or practice administrator.

But be very careful about how you phrase your questions and how you present yourself to them as they can be an important part of the hiring process.

When my kids were young, I used to make it clear when I interviewed that I am a single mom, and I have a custody agreement I have to follow. My philosophy is to be upfront and honest in an interview. If they know your capabilities and limitations, there won't be any surprises later on. The type of people you want to work with will understand your situation. If they don't, this isn't the place for you. Just move on to the next opportunity. There will be more jobs out there, or you will create one!

When I took a part-time cardiology position that was advertised for twenty hours a week, I worked with the HR manager to work out being available for two ten-hour days. On my first day, the cardiologist and I were talking about the schedule, and when he realized I was doing two ten-hour days and not five four hour days, he got furious. Obviously, there had been some miscommunication as there was no way I could have made that type of schedule work for me and he wanted someone there five days a week. What a lovely welcome to my fist cardiology gig! I had arranged childcare, and turned down several other opportunities. The mistake on my part was negotiating with the HR department, who did not ask for his input. Yet another reason to know your true employer.

Lesson learned. Always get your schedule, whatever is essential or promised to you, written down on paper as an agreement before accepting any position. Most practices send out an offer letter, simply ask for all of the agreed hours, benefits, salary, and incentives in writing. I know it may take a little longer and may not be something they are used to if it is a smaller practice, but it will be worth it and give you peace of mind knowing what you and they agreed upon.

So many practices are used to this as they have multiple physicians they have hired, and to do this, they have to have a contract with specific terms. If they are not willing to do this, you may need to rethink working with them. Many PAs these days have contracts with their hospitals and organizations where they are employed. If you have one, make sure you go through the details. Take your time and understand the terms of the contract, or have a lawyer review its terms and conditions. Always review the insurance coverage and what happens after you leave the position. This will definitely save you some anxiety in the future.

A great piece of advice we received in PA school is to always think long and hard about working for a practice in which the physician is married to another staff member or practice manager. This situation can be challenging to work with and can make for some awkward moments around the office. That's all I have to say about that. You can figure out the rest from here and decide what risks you are willing to take. I'm just throwing it out there to let you know it is not uncommon.

Consider shadowing someone at the practice where you are interviewing. Volunteer to come in for a morning, afternoon, or entire day to see how the practice is run and see if the opportunity is a good fit for you. This will allow you to observe and ask questions in a less anxious environment. I have done it with a few positions, and it has made a difference in my expectations going into a new job.

The Grass Can Actually Be Greener

While in PA school, so many of us have ideas of exactly what type of practice and specialty we would like to be in. Some of my fellow classmates even had jobs waiting for them when they graduated. I thought I would likely work in cardiothoracic surgery. However, I have not ever worked in CTS. I have had several offers, but it just never really worked out. I never thought that I would have worked in cardiology for nine years, or in neurosurgery, or for the VA for that matter. I simply saw each opportunity as an excellent way to learn a new skill set and broaden my strengths.

If you haven't read *Who Moved My Cheese* by Spencer Johnson, you should. It is such a fantastic book about not staying in a stagnant situation because you are scared of what is next. In his book, he says, "Smell the cheese often, so you know when it is getting old." And, "When you move beyond your fear, you will feel free."

Sometimes, we stay in an unsatisfactory work environment. Other times, our favorite coworkers move on, the dynamic changes and the environment we are working in seems un-healthy. Don't be afraid to try something new, broaden your skills, and learn a different aspect of medicine. See it as a chal-lenge and an opportunity to become more marketable and valu-able. And the experience of learning something new and getting to work with different people is always fun. As I stated earlier, I moved over to neurosurgery. I was terrified to change and could not manage to see over the horizon. I had been in cardiology for nine years and loved my patients, but the environment had changed. Coworkers had come and gone, and I was becoming more and more frustrated due to circumstances I could not control. I made a leap of faith to a different specialty, and it was one of the best decisions ever. Who you work with each day is important. Do not stay in a position you are not feel fulfilled. Take a chance and bet on something new.

A friend and mentor of mine once said, "Rachel, always choose what's going to lead to more opportunities." Look for a job where you will have the most opportunities that are important to you. Opportunities might entail a position that will allow you to become knowledgeable in a specific specialty that provides outstanding training. You can quickly become an expert in that field. You can be the one at meetings giving lectures. Or you may look for a position where you can do research and publish papers. Or you may look for a situation in which you can get involved in administrative duties and leadership within your organization. Again, you have to figure out where you want to be and what you want to be doing in order to figure out what these opportunities may look like for you specifically.

When I worked for Medtronic, I accompanied one of the nurse practitioners out to California to meet a fellow NP who was an expert in her field. She was running a cancer pain clinic for patients with intrathecal pain pumps. She was incredible, and we both learned so much from meeting with her. She and the physician she worked with had come up with extraordinary protocols and treatment plans that were effective for their patients. She, of course, was paid very well for sharing her time and her expertise with us. That could be you. You can be speaking at conferences and furthering research to better patients' lives, not only in your own practice but others' practices as well.

I was divorced for about 12 years before I got remarried. During that time, I dated many people, and if you are out in the dating world, then you know how crazy it can be in your late 30's early 40's. Quite often, I called my friend Cheryl to tell her my stories and complain about the weirdos and their issues. One day she said to me in her very matter-of-fact southern drawl, "Rachel, everyone has shit. It's just whose shit do you want to put up with?" This is so true in both relationships and in jobs. Every position you consider will have some negative aspects and things that you just do not like. Ask yourself if you are willing to put up with those negative issues, and you just might want to, because the positive things about the job far outweigh the negative.

You may be in a small town with limited PA positions, and your job options are limited. Consider those limitations as something positive. You can make the most of any situation if you have the right attitude. Keep an open mind, and always seek ways to advance your knowledge. Look for opportunities in every challenge you face. The smaller the practice, the more you will learn the different aspects of office operations, practice marketing, billing, coding, and people management. Maybe you want to open your own business someday, take this as an opportunity for on-the-job training.

Interviewing and choosing a PA job is an exciting time. Make sure you are getting what you want out of your career. Realize the most important decision about your job is that you have to make sure the position is a good fit for you, ok, a great fit for you. You have to research each opportunity and interview anyone who will talk with you about it. If you have several choices, choose the best for you, your family, and your career goals. You spend a tremendous amount of time at work. Do what you love, and you will be successful at it!

Chapter 4

Helpful Tips for Working Well With Your Attending Physician/Physicians

"It is literally true that you can succeed best and quickest by helping others to succeed."

—*Napoleon Hill*
Self-help author

Now that you have landed that stellar new job, it is time to get down to business. Being purpose-driven in relationships with your physicians, patients, and staff will prove to be fundamental in a successful career. Let's start by working on building an excellent supervising PA/physician relationship. When you seek to understand who you are working with and what drives them, you will have a more cohesive team approach. The exciting news is that you will not only be building strong working relationships; you will cultivate invaluable friendships throughout your career as well. Your physicians will be your mentors, friends, and allies. You will be an asset to their practice and a champion for their patients. You want them to trust you with every part of their practice. You are a representation of each physician you work with. You are the frontline.

Getting To Know You

The key to working with your physicians is to make sure they see you as a valuable asset and a vital part of their practice. Thus, you need to figure out your relationship with each of them. When you first start working with your physician, make sure you analyze how they work. Go with them when they visit their patients and observe how they interact with them. I tend to remember almost word-for-word some of the things my doctors say to patients. Of course, they had some years to perfect it, but I promise that your doctor won't mind it if you use the same wording. Imitation is a form of flattery, right? It takes time, wisdom, and understanding to get your wording straight on diseases, procedures, and medications. Wording is so important so that not only will your patients understand what you are saying, but they will also realize the importance of what you are asking them to do.

You will be able to learn a great deal by observing how the physicians treat and respond to their patients. What is their attitude like? How is their demeanor? Are they approachable with their patients and staff? How are they treating you? Have they set clear expectations? When you are seeing patients alongside them, how do they respond when you ask questions or interact with the patients? Definitely be cognizant of these things and pick up on their body language. You have to figure out if this is going to be a friendly type of work relationship or a structured business-only interaction when you are working with them. It would be great to know those things before working with someone, but you just can't pick up on everything during an interview. You will be able to gain so much knowledge in your observations of them and how they treat their patients, the staff, and you. Use this information to your advantage.

Where To Start

They need to see that you are enthusiastic and willing to learn, especially in the beginning, when they will be teaching you how they like things to operate around the office, hospital and operating room. Ask them what they recommend for you to read; what conferences to go to, what apps they are using in their practice. Make sure you take some notes on your phone to make sure you remember.

When I first started in neurosurgery, I was more than over-whelmed with the learning curve I had in front of me. I had no idea of where to even start. I was talking with one of the doctors I was working with and his suggestion was to get the *Handbook of Neurosurgery*, read through it, and learn from it. I did not get through all of it at one time, but I read over and over again the critical diseases and treatments we ran into in our practice. It was beneficial and focused my attention on one educational area. Starting out, I didn't need to go from journal to book or website to website, all I needed was to start with something easy enough and work my way from there.

Simply ask what they want you to do to get to where you need to be. Do not try to guess, as they may have one easy solution for you to get started. Once you are up and rolling, you will know what direction you need to follow.

I would also speak with each person your provider works with regularly and learn the ins and outs of how things are done. Take time with the appointment scheduler, the procedure/sur-gery scheduler, the medical assistants, nurses and whoever else is making the practice run. Ask how the physician prefers things to be handled and learn as much as you can from them. Use them as a huge resource and you will not have to bug your physician with all of your questions. This will allow you to work with all of the staff, and they will recognize that you are there to help things run as smoothly as possible. I guarantee that when your providers know that you are taking time to learn, understand, and master the practice and how operations work, they will im-mediately start trusting you. And once you see what is and isn't working, you can make some suggestions to help things operate more smoothly.

Sometimes, when you start working with your physician and you do not understand why they are doing something in a particular way or if they forget to teach you, just ask them, "From a teaching perspective, can you help me understand that decision?" When you ask him or her, inquiring from a teaching perspective, it does not seem like you are questioning them and their methods, you are merely seeking to learn. I will even say, "Okay, I'm confused. (This is totally not an uncommon statement from me) I thought you usually did this, but now you are doing something else, can you help me understand?" This line of questioning might also help in case you disagree with your physician about a decision. Try to be as non-confrontational as possible.

It is essential to understand their nuisances and the key drivers of their decisions. What is right for one patient is not for the next per se. I also think kindly questioning them, and coming from a learning perspective shows that you are paying attention, seeking to understand, wishing to incorporate their reasoning for doing things into your own practice. This is why you have to understand their 'why.' See a pattern here? If you understand why they do the things they do, then it will be easier to put it into practice.

If you are going to question anyone's medical decisions, I would suggest speaking up only after you have the literature and knowledge of proper practice to back you up. I promise you at some point, as you come to know best practices and put them to use, you will sometimes question those you work with. It happens. Coming from an honest and kind mindset when questioning a physician or another PA, it might help them refocus. They also might see it as an indication to explain better just what it is that they are doing. Even if their way is the best way, it may give them pause to consider explaining this reasoning more clearly in their documentation. If you don't understand it clearly, how is a jury ever going to understand their decision making?

All physicians practice differently. It is a fact. They may all be focused on doing what is best for their patients, but there can be a thousand ways to get there or there could be three. You do the math. So you may have this dilemma quite frequently. If you work with multiple doctors, you might want to take notes at the beginning of how they like things done, especially when their name is on the chart along with yours. Some differences are just technical, like wanting all their patients called regardless if labs come back normal or abnormal. And some just want the abnormal labs called back. You have to find a way that works best for everyone. You don't want to do the same thing five different ways. Ask and address issues upfront. Don't let the sun go down on your confusion.

Your doctors will always want to know how the other providers practice medicine. If you are coming from another practice within the same specialty—especially a teaching institution—you will get a ton of questions. This will allow you to train your physicians—particularly if they are slow to catch up on best practices. Yes, those folks are out there too, and it is not always the older physicians that are the issue. Sometimes it is the younger, arrogant ones that cannot be taught a single thing. Be mindful of how you address this, and please don't be that person that judgingly says every other day, "Well, this is how we did it at Mayo."

My children's grandfather taught me a useful phrase that I used to roll my eyes at, but have come to adopt as my own. It goes something like, "Based on _____, May I make a suggestion?" I love this, and it certainly might help you help others in your office. It allows them an out if they don't want helpful ideas and it allows you and in if they do! Find something that is not too pushy, but gets your idea across. There will always be those who are averse to trying anything new. These folks are easy to spot and ignore. Don't waste your time or energy.

If you want to be well-received and thoroughly listened to, make sure to take time to observe, ask a lot of questions to clarify, and make sure you have all of the information you need before you come up with helpful solutions or suggestions.

Linda, Honey, Listen To Me!

When you are reviewing a patient with your physician, sometimes they do not listen to everything you say. It has happened with every physician I have ever worked with. Basically, they are just not paying attention. I know this has not just happened to me. Right? They are thinking about the patient they just examined, a text they got from their mistress, or something entirely unrelated to work. We all have been there.

How often do I zone out when my kids are talking to me? Okay, they will tell you I do it all of the time. Your physicians are no different. I have gotten responses from physicians that were completely off base. They will ask me to run a regular exercise stress test on a man who does not have any legs when I have just informed them of the fact that they were blown off by an IED in Iraq. (Should I tell you that I just typed out IUD instead of IED? Now that would be an interesting story, a story that might just deserve its own book). I've had doctors tell me to use a particular medicine when I just briefed them that the patient tried that one and ended up getting loopy on it and ended up waking up in a dumpster. Surely, things like this have happened to you?

When this happens, know that you are not alone; just take a long deep breath, or three, before reminding them of what you just told them. Put some emphasis on what's important. Make sure you are being brief enough in your description and that everything you are telling them is pertinent for decision making. They may not appreciate or need to hear about how the patient's grandson owns a gym down the street, and he and his wife are bodybuilders. (Save that gym discount for you. Remember, you got to start taking care of yourself.) Just recap, retell, and refocus their attention. Knowing damned-well what you already said, kindly say, "Oh, I'm sorry, did I mention that he has no legs?" Take the blame, rephrase what you said, send flares up or just do something creative to get their attention so you can take care of the patient. I will sometimes put my hand-written notes in front of them so they can see, listen, and read at the same time. Get as many of their senses going at one time so you can get your job done, and they can get back to texting or shopping on Cabela's website.

I Have A Question

Is it just me, or does it bug you too that some people have to announce that they have a question before asking their question? Or, better yet, when they inform you that they have a quick question? Yes, they may have a quick question, but the answer you have to give is much longer and time-consuming than you would prefer. Just a pet peeve, I suppose. Anyway, I believe it is important to ask questions to your doctors when you cannot find the answer anywhere else. Asking a ton of questions is sometimes, or a lot of times, ridiculously irritating. If from nowhere else, I certainly have learned this from having two very inquisitive children.

What I found helpful is to write my questions down, so I have several at a time to ask, but then I ask them infrequently as not to bug them too much. I also like to diversify. I will ask one physician a few questions and then a different doctor another set of questions and then the NP a separate list. That way, I am getting everything answered, just not all by the same person. Timing is important. Definitely read the room and know when it is a good time. If you have to ask if it is a good time, it probably isn't.

You also have to work with your physician on how they like to interact. If you are in the operating room and your physician is throwing things and yelling at the staff, it may not be the best time to bring up your question on renewing Mr. Epstein's Viagra prescription.

You could try asking these: Do you want me to save my questions for the end of the day/first thing in the morning? Do you want me to text you throughout the day with questions? When you ask to know, they understand your need and eagerness to learn and do the best job possible. Sit down, and set your expectations upfront, so you can build a strong foundation together to treat your patients. Know your doctor, know their preferences.

Always seek to understand.

It's Not You. It's Me

As I mentioned earlier, I used to work with intrathecal drug delivery systems, also known as pain pumps. Part of working with the pumps is to calculate the dosage to be given, get it from the pump, through the tubing and into the patient. It can take a while for the drug to reach the patient unless you calculate a bolus of medication to make it through the tubing quickly and then distribute it as needed. I thought I had everything right, but when the doctor told me the next morning, after the surgery, that the patient wasn't feeling better, I wondered why. I went over my notes and calculations and realized I had messed up. I had under-dosed the patient, and it was my fault. So, I immediately went into his office and fessed up.

What I could have done is fixed the problem, never said a word and carried on about my work. But I couldn't do it. He didn't get mad. He did not get angry. He knew that I never had to say a word to him and could have taken care of the patient on my won. He told me right then and there how much respect he had for me for coming to him and taking the blame for the under-calculation. Ever since then, we've had a fantastic working relationship.

If you make a mistake, take care of it quickly, and own up to it as soon as you realize it. Go let the right people know and do whatever you can to make things right. It stinks, it's embarrassing, and it could prove harmful to your patient or others, but it is the right thing to do. You will gain more respect by being honest, taking the blame, correcting what you can, and moving on. Don't forget to forgive yourself. Learn what to do better next time and let it go.

Grunt Work

You will find that when you work with a practice in which there are many procedures to be done, your physician will most likely want to be performing procedures and surgeries rather than being in clinic. I see many practices in which the physicians only see consults in clinic and the remainder of their time is spent in procedures and surgery. In case you don't know, this is where the big bucks are. Your physician and practice can charge and be reimbursed far more for a procedure than they can a clinic visit. So while they are busy making sure they can pay for next month's mortgage, boat and Super Bowl tickets, it also means that they will leave some of the not so thrilling work for you to do—like discharge summaries. These are definitely not one of my favorite responsibilities.

Keep in mind that it is their job to delegate. You are the physician assistant. You were hired to be helpful and profitable to them. Even if some of the items on the to-do list for the day suck, it makes you appreciate the other 99 things on your list that you do like. You have to take the good with the bad. There is much work to be done, and they trust you to get the necessary items accomplished with a fairly pleasant demeanor. If they are delegating something to you that you can delegate to somebody else, by all means, do so. However, some things can only be done by you or your physician. Take your time, do your best, and forget the rest.

Level Up

When you are done with the work you are not so excited about, start thinking about what you can do to add value to your practice and move to the next level of customer satisfaction and state-of-the-art care. Start learning things that your physician does not know about but needs to, in order for you make yourself more valuable. Are you getting a new EMR? Become the expert quickly. Are there new hospital procedures/protocols/compliance rules and regulations? Go to the meetings, and learn all of these things. Volunteer to go above and beyond.

Take the initiative to see what needs to be done and take care of it. Do some research, come up with a proposal. Look into what some of the well-respected practices are doing. Look into that new equipment you have wanted to get. Go out of your way to make the doctors and other providers aware of what an asset you are. Don't tell them, show them. Show them with your work ethic, your attitude, your forward-thinking, and your commitment to solving problems. They will see your value and necessity within the organization, and those extra measures are what make you and your job indispensable.

Remember that this is a business and this business is there to make money. You are their employee, and you are there to help the practice financially and to treat your patients with the best care possible.

Make It Your Own

Sometimes you get the opportunity to work with many physicians, nurse practitioners and PAs in your practice. Study the best practices from them and incorporate them into your own practice. Find who the best educator is in your practice and learn how they interact with their patients. Understand how they explain difficult concepts, diseases, medicines, procedures, and surgeries. Use their knowledge and wisdom and begin to educate your patients in the same manner.

Some providers may be better at knowing the literature and practice guidelines. These people might not be the best educators or be even remotely good at having any kind of bedside manners. Sometimes there are providers within your practice who are better at administrative roles. See how they work and learn from their business acumen. It truly is your job to learn from the best and then adopt these golden nuggets into your clinical practice. This is where heart of medicine is. This is the art of medicine. You need to wear several hats in order to be an excellent fit for the practice, and the best you can be for your patients.

Purposefully learning from those who are consistently reliable in certain areas will help you be fantastic at your job. As you learn more, your physicians will look to your knowledge and leadership to learn from you. I have seen it time and again with PAs I have worked with. You are the approachable one, the one who is learning from the representatives, and the one who is constantly improving yourself. Before you know it, other providers will seek out your help and knowledge in every area of your practice.

Working with your physicians will be one of the most important daily interactions you have. Seeking to learn, understand their needs and desires for you as their PA, and providing outstanding care for patients is of utmost importance. Get this right, find a good physician that practices best-in-class medicine and treats patients well. Seek to find the right working environment for you and your skill set. Enjoy where you work and who you work for. Become their best asset so they will never want to let you leave. Be willing to do the work they don't want to take on. Seek to improve their business practice and efficiency. Help take them to the next level. Become everything your physicians are not willing to be, but need to be, in order to be successful. Work hard every day to help make your doctors and your hospital or practice look good.

Be purposeful and indispensable!

Chapter 5

Helpful Tips for Working Well With Your Patients

They may forget your name, but they will never forget how you made them feel.

—*Maya Angelou*
Author

Working with patients has always been the best part of my job and possibly yours too. That's why we got into medicine, right? There are not too many areas where people thank you for doing, asking, and telling the most horrific things to them.

You pull out their ingrown toe. "Thank you."

You stick a needle into their abdomen to do a paracentesis. "Thank you."

You stick colonoscopes, speculums, nasogastric tubes, and all kinds of other instrumentation to examine body parts they aren't keen on sharing with others. "Thank you."

You tell them they are dying, but before you walk out the door. "Thank you."

You tell them they are obese, their cholesterol is high, and they need to exercise, lose weight, and stop smoking. You have completely hurt their feelings and pride, but, "Thank you."

How crazy! I love that—for the most part—patients are gracious and grateful. In medicine, we are thanked every day by our patients. This is such an exciting reward. Sometimes it might be difficult to get a "thank you" or "good job" out of the people you work with. But know that when you are doing your best for your patients, you will get praise and accolades from them. Remember, they are the actual customer you are truly working for.

When I was pregnant with my first child, some of my patients were more excited than I was about me having a baby. One patient actually had his wife knit a blanket, jacket, and booties for my son. It was one of the sweetest and most memorable gifts I have ever received, and of course, twenty years later, I still cherish those precious items.

I have received the most incredible words of encouragement and gratitude. Out of the goodness of their heart and gardens, I have received letters, rosaries, flowers, specialty peaches and oranges, and handmade necklaces and a couple of bowls of amazing gumbo just to name a few. Each time I am reminded of how lucky and blessed I am to have such amazing people in my life.

These patients are precious and need to be cared for in the best way possible. You just might be the only light they may see in a day. So it is very important to treat them with the honor and respect they deserve.

When YOU Talk, Patients Listen

When I first got out training, I felt I had a strong foundation and a pretty good recall for the basics of what I was taught.

My sister came to Houston to visit me with her two children. Houston is the vacation Hot Spot for mosquitos. Her then three-year-old daughter got a mosquito bite on her cheek that swelled up fairly nicely, kind of like a huge zit that you used to get on your face, like right before you were going out with that special someone you were truly excited about. My sister completely freaked out and told me she was going to the emergency room immediately as there must be something imminently wrong. Madeline was fine—breathing well, not crying, not itching, not really too swollen, eating well, drinking well etc. I simply said, "Rhonda, they're probably going to look at her bite, tell you to give her some Benadryl and then they are going to send you home, so really, I wouldn't waste my time or money." Obviously, that went over like a brick and she packed up her kids and headed straight for the ER. Several hours later, she came home after stopping by Walgreens to get some more Benadryl.

And this is one of the numerable instances where my family has not taken my advice. So if your family does not listen to your advice either, just know that you are not alone. It happens to all of us. But, eventually, your family will realize that you know what you are talking about and that you could have saved them lots of money, time, and "noteworthy" ER visits.

Your family might not always follow your advice, but your patients usually do!

I'll just say it like this. **Know what you are talking about!** Patients *do* listen to the advice and the explanations you give to them. This is why it's critical to really know what you are explaining to them and put explanations into words they can easily understand. If you didn't know the word before PA school, maybe you shouldn't use it to explain to them what is going on. Borborygmi is not a household term.

Take time as you are talking, make sure you are a little more slowed in your speech and you enunciate clearly and make good eye contact.

Within cardiology, I often found that my patients would come in and tell me that they were told that after their cardiac catheterization that the doctor's told them "There's nothing we can do for you." This often left them thinking, "Okay, I guess I can just go home and die of a heart attack at some point in time." When in reality, they would only have one or two blockages of 20–30% or so that required no procedure, stent, or surgical intervention to correct that level of blockage. There really was nothing that they could do to open up the artery, however, the doctors failed to mention, that the artery was not at the point to even need intervention. The patients were left thinking that they had horrible disease and there was nothing that could actually be done, instead of leaving the procedure understanding that they do have some disease but it is not at the point of needing anything done at this time. There is a big difference here.

It is imperative to take the time to properly educate, speak clearly, and answer questions. Think about drawing a diagram for a visual aid.

I have learned to add in a qualifier when talking to my patients and it goes something like this.

"At this time, you do have coronary artery disease, however, it does not require any intervention or procedures or surgeries. The arteries have minimal blockage. However, it does not mean that down the line you will not need to do x, y, or z. At this time we will need to treat your condition like this, however, in the future you may need x, y or z if we cannot medically keep your disease from progressing."

Statements like this let them know that you are working with them to treat their condition the best you can and if needed down the line, there might be something that will be recommended. However, if nothing can be done, by all means let them know and be specific about what their expectations should be of their disease process and likelihood of progression.

We may presume the provider that came before us did all the patient education for us. Have you ever assumed this? Please don't. Ask the patient what their understanding of their disease is. This just might be one of the most important questions to ask your patients. It will let you know the true level of understanding that the patient and family have, and what you need to do to further their level of knowledge. The better you educate your patients and family, the less often they will call the office. They will be more compliant with instructions and the risk of more frequent visits, hospitalizations, and readmissions will likely go down.

Just An Expression

One day I was on hospital rounds with one of the physicians I did not work with regularly. English is his second language, and he was educating a patient about having a cardiac catheterization and echocardiogram. He was trying to tell the patient we would get some tests done so we could figure out what was going on with him and evaluate a cause for his symptoms. What he meant to say was we will nail down a reason for your symptoms, but what he said was, "We'll put the final nail in the coffin." You should have seen the look on the patient's face. It was priceless and I'm pretty sure he was leaning over to get his shoes on to make a quick escape. Maybe this isn't the best to use when your patients are facing their own mortality. Not only should you know how to educate your patients, but also have your expressions down pat as well. If you get a strange look from your patients, maybe it's time to think about what you just said and see if it seems appropriate for the situation. I can't tell you how many times I've said something like, "I'm dying to hear about it!" That's always a great one with our geriatric patients who lose friends just about every week. We all do some silly things and say things that we wish we could take back or say a little differently. None of us want to offend anyone. It's a learning process for all of us to be intentional with every word we are using with our patients.

Know Your Limits

So now that we've talked about how much our patients listen to us and the importance of genuinely knowing what we are talking about, let's talk about knowing what we don't know. To put it plainly, I have found it is not worth bullshitting my way through any conversation with any patient or patient's family member, your physician, or anyone else. Don't you remember being on rounds with your fellow students and someone trying to sound way smarter than they were or making it sound like they totally asked the patient about a symptom and it is clear as day that they never even thought to ask them that? You knew they seemed ridiculous and were full of it.

Admitting that I don't know what I don't know is one of the critical lessons I learned in PA school, and it has earned me so much respect from my patients. Don't be afraid to say you don't know or you didn't ask. It shows honesty and integrity. We all mess up and forget to ask key questions. It happens and is an important part of the learning process.

I'll be the first to admit it. I sometimes just don't have all the answers. Ask my twenty and eighteen-year-olds. One of the two most frequent phrases they heard from me when they were growing up is, "please chew with your mouth closed." And "I don't know, why don't you look it up?" Why is it that they always ask you questions about things you know nothing of anyways?

When I was working in cardiology and would be getting ready to go in with a new consultation, and I saw "dizziness" as the reason for consultation, I would just roll my eyes and then gear up. I don't know many people who see that particular chief complaint and get excited about it. It is a challenging term and sometimes exasperating to figure out what is going on with the patient. Usually, by the time the patient had gotten to me in cardiology, he or she was utterly frustrated, bent out of shape, and looking for answers and looking for answers right NOW.

I had to learn to sit down with them, really listen for a good long time without interrupting and then usually say, "I don't know why this is happening." However, I follow that up with "Let's work together, do some testing, and then let's get to the bottom of this. If I can't help figure out what is going on, I'll try to get you to someone who can. I know you have had this for a while, and you are frustrated by these symptoms. I may not have an answer immediately, but again, let's work on it together." Then I usually tell them the first steps and then if no explanation for their symptoms, the second steps, and so on.

I cannot tell you how much patients appreciate it when you just say, "I don't know, " and then you tell them you'll work with them the best you can to figure out an explanation. If you can admit that you don't know something to your patients, then when you do speak with them and educate them on other topics, they will have the utmost confidence in you!

After working in cardiology for nine years and changing over to neurosurgery, I was all too familiar with saying, "I'm not quite sure, let me speak with Dr. Wolter, and I'll be right back in." Neurosurgery is a creature of its own. I didn't know how long the hospitalization was going to be for a fusion, or how long for the patient would be expected to be off work, or how long I should write for a handicap parking placard, or if the doctor is going to go ahead and write for a year's supply of Percocet. These are little questions, but takes time when you are going into a new specialty. There is no way PA training can prepare you for these questions, nor are you going to read them in any books. They are on-the-job specific and take a lot of time and repetition before you get it down and feel confident in your role. It takes time and know it is ok for you to say that you just don't know the answer.

I find that when patients are getting information from you and you've been talking to them and educating them and answering their questions during an exam. Then you get to one where you just don't know the answer to it, they then think "ok, she has been honest all along, and now she's admitting that she doesn't know something and she's going to get the answer to it, she must have been telling the truth on all the other stuff."

And sometimes, you don't know the answer, and you may be in the clinic by yourself. It's ok to simply tell the patient that you don't have the answer, but that you will try to get it and then get back with them once you do. You're probably saying, "But I'm a PA. I'm supposed to know what to do...." We cannot all be good at every aspect of practicing medicine. I have spent the majority of my career in outpatient care. Even after 16 years of medicine, if you give me an emergency, I will not know what to do necessarily. I'm just hoping that someone is there for me to yell, "call 911 and get and AED!" and that a crash cart happens to be around the corner with someone who knows what they are doing right next to it.

Several years ago I was driving down the highway and I saw a man purposely job off the bridge right in front of me. I was alone and kept thinking, "Really? I'm on my way to the antique mall (something of which I rarely ever do...anymore). Did this guy really just do this? Now I have to stop. What in the world am I going to do? Having a patient jump off a bridge right in front of me was never the scenario they had on any of my tests." I remained calm. In the beginning, I did not know what to do other than call 911, and figure out the ABC's…but calmness in the situation helps. And things do start to kick in, eventually! Unfortunately, for the gentleman I came across, I don't think anything I could have done could have helped him.

The more I learn about medicine, the more I realize I cannot be good at all aspects of it. For me, it has been nice to specialize and become an expert in my specialty. If you are a primary care PA, be the best you can. If you are a nephrology PA, be the best at that specialty. Focus in that area and be determined to be the best within it.

A phrase that I have heard many a physician say when asked about other aspects of medicine is this: "That's not my area of expertise, but here are my suggestions"…and they either send the patient to someone who can help them, or back to the PCP who can redirect them to appropriate care.

Know your limits, do your best and know that there is no way that you can be great at all aspects of medicine. There are experts in every medical arena for a reason. They dedicate their life to knowing everything about that one small area. Don't beat yourself up over not knowing everything. Be the best you can be where you currently are.

Extra, Extra, Read All About it

When I was about ten, my mom took me to the doctor for some breast tenderness I was having. I know this sound crazy, but hear me out. So, I am at the office and tell the nurse, Flo, all my boob issues and she hands me a gown, which was really just a paper grocery sack of some sort that looked more like a vest than a gown. After some type of strange examination in which my family doctor examined my breasts, he handed me two small booklets to read. These little gems had all of the fun language and pictures to help educate me on what to expect about getting my period. I had just got felt up by him, so I was pretty excited that he gave me a little memento to remember our visit as I walked out the door.

I think by this time, most girls know what will be coming down from the nether regions? I don't know, the 1980s were a long time ago. But what I do know is that I looked through those booklets several times with interest and confusion. There were some interesting pictures, and both told me about something I had never heard of before, the period pad belt. Do you even know what this is? It seemed like one of the most horrible and completely uncomfortable contraptions ever. You mean, when I get my period and am bleeding all over the place, I'm going to wear a belt made of what looks like burlap underneath my clothes to keep a pad in place? What the hell is going on? I had never seen my older sister or my mom with anything that looked anywhere near like the odd pictures in the book.

What was everyone hiding from me? Where were the pictures of tampons and how to put one of those things in? I had seen those before in the cabinets and heard my older friends speak of those. Don't even get me started on how my friend Heather and I tried to get my first one of those plastic and cotton bullets in so I could go swimming at the pool with her. However, through a little research while doing this book, apparently the period pad belt was invented like, a long time ago. It was outdated and replaced with the lovely adhesive pads, which we know and love today, back in the 1970s. My doctor was kind, trying to give me a little information, especially since my mom would never have thought to discuss my period. But his information was entirely out of date, almost traumatizing and indeed extremely confusing to my ten year old self. Have you ever received or given someone irrelevant literature?

Needless to say, you might want to keep up to date and read through your patient literature that your office has before your patient comes in expecting to get their own period pad belt.

Patient literature will be one of the best ways to educate your patients and their loved ones. These brochures can be very educational and have great visual aids. In addition, I have found that some of the pharmaceutical and device representatives have resources that can be helpful for patients too. Just ask them to bring some in. Not all of the patient literature they give will be just about the product they sell. You can also download patient literature from so many sites to print off and hand out. I use UP-TO-DATE the most frequently and will often print out the information for my patients while they are in the office.

Anytime I have changed specialties, I would get all the brochures our offices had in the lobby and in patient rooms, and I would read them. Then I would look through a few of my favorite reference books like Harrison's to refresh my memory on disease states and then I would move on to the specialty books in a step wise process, getting into more and more details.

Once you're well educated and comfortable with your knowledge, you can inform and educate your patients even better. Remember, you don't want to give too much information because patients tend to get overwhelmed. Start with the basics, and give a little more with each follow up visit.

Be familiar with websites, apps, and organizations that are patient-friendly and who are trustworthy. There are plenty of sites founded by reliable organizations to send your patients to.

It would be helpful to have a handout available with all of your regular recommendations, so you are not constantly writing down the same information.

The More, The Merrier

Have you ever walked in with one of your patients and there is absolutely nowhere for you to sit or stand because they have so many people in the room with them? I have found that some providers get a little irritated when multiple family members are in the room when they come in for a consultation or follow up. See it as an opportunity. An opportunity for numerous sets of ears to listen to what you have to say and to encourage the patient with the directions you have given. I find that I receive fewer phone calls and, again, better compliance, if I have a patient family member or caregiver present to help remind the patient of the things we talk about.

Remember that as you talk with your patients, you may be repeating the same lecture and healthy lifestyle speech all day every day and it may make complete sense to you. For your patient, this is the first time they have ever heard this information and it is about them and they may be overwhelmed and scared. Be patient, be kind, and slow down a little.

Two Ears, One Mouth

How good of a listener are you? Are you focused on what you are hearing from your patients, or do you walk in the door with a plan based on the chief complaint your medical assistant gave you, determined you know what to do without even hearing for yourself what your patient has to say? Are you taking time to listen to what they are saying, how they say it, and observing their body language as they talk with you? There are instances when I have walked in the door with paperwork and consults completed before I even spoke to my patient. I think I am saving time and being efficient and that I have everything under control. I can also tell you that after listening and hearing what is truly going on, I have thrown my original plan out the window and have come up with a different plan altogether more times than not.

Listening to your patients is the best skill you can continue to master throughout your career.

Are we truly listening to our patients and giving them time to get their thoughts out before we start expressing our own opinions? Dr. Jerome Groopman, the author of *How Doctors Think*, states that doctors interrupt their patients within 18 seconds of the start of their conversation. This is unacceptable for us as providers. We have to be respectful and listen to our patients to find out what they truly need. Our patients deserve our full concentration and attention. Your patients want to be heard. I use phrases like, "I understand" and "I hear you" quite a bit to give them reassurance that I am completely hearing what they are telling me.

I worked for the VA for over twelve years. For the majority of those twelve years, I typed all my notes, ordered all the consults, labs, procedures, and tests for my patients by myself. I was a one-woman show and had to take full responsibility for every aspect of each patient's care. There was no one else to do it. I usually had the patient in the room with me while I was ordering everything and would ask them to give me a few minutes while I put orders in. For some reason, it was during this time, where I needed to concentrate, that patients got uncomfortable with the silence and started talking. I would learn all kinds of things. Sometimes it would be more about their symptoms. It might have been about their social issues or even about what happened to them twenty years ago when they were in the service.

If you want to learn about your patients, simply stay quiet. It is incredible what you can discover and how this information can help you treat the patients or understand where they are coming from. At the very least, you'll end up with an entertaining story to tell in your book later.

Within the practice of cardiology, you can imagine that many patients have erectile dysfunction. It has been many a time in my silence and typing away at the keyboard that the patient says, "Hey, Rachel, do you think you can prescribe me some of that Viagra?" or "I'm afraid of dying." or, "I just found out I have a son I did not know about." They have all kinds of questions, all types of concerns that need to be addressed. During these times of silence, patients will ask questions that they are often afraid to ask at any other time.

I will even be in the midst of speaking to patients and realize that I am not getting the root of their problem what so ever, so I will purposefully cause an awkward moment of silence just to get them to speak a little more. Trust me; it will work to your advantage.

Keep in mind that there could be an additional gain from patients having appointments with you. Several years ago, I was seeing a patient in the clinic, and I could not figure out what was going on with him as his statements were contradictory. I was trying to tell him once more what I was hearing so that I could figure out what tests I needed to order and document his symptoms accurately. I sat there for a moment, waiting for the computer to boot up or something of that nature, and finally, he says to me, "I'm really here because I need to have my disability increased so I can make more money to pay my bills each month." Aha, Aha! I wasn't confused after all. He was the one being confusing because he had no idea what to say to get what he needed out of the appointment. I think when he heard me repeat in his own words of what he had said, he understood the ridiculousness of his claims, and he felt compelled to tell me the truth. This brings to attention another good point: telling the patient back what you are hearing them say, so they can try to make sense of their own words and clarify. I will often say, "So this is what I am hearing you say... is this correct?"

Sometimes the care you provide for someone's physical health may be a small part of why they came to their appointment. Some patients only want to have someone safe they can talk to. Keeping this in mind for our older patients is very important. This may be the only social outing they have for the whole week. These patients might not have anyone else who cares or looks after them. So if you find yourself wondering why you do not understand the real complaints or needs of your patient, or when symptoms and time-frames just don't make any sense, keep in mind that the patient could be there for some other reason. Sometimes patients are not safe at home. Make sure you can have a private conversation with your patient and do not be afraid to ask if your patient feels safe in his or her home environment.

Listening to what your patients are saying and not saying and how they are giving you non-verbal cues is essential in being successful in your career. Stop. Look. Listen. Maybe this should be the second golden rule?

Pen to Paper

During your training, did you sit and listen to lectures because you knew you would retain all the information the speaker was giving you? Did the speaker just talk and not have any slides or visual aids? Speakers usually had visual aids, and most of the time, you were probably taking notes furiously. Why are having PowerPoints and taking notes so helpful? Uhhh, you remember things better if you see, hear, and write them down.

Your patients are no different from you. They need all those tools to understand and remember what is going on and what they need to do. Some of your patients and family members will be writing down some of what you are saying, but most will not. I keep a pad of Post-Its® with me or write down on their printed off medication list the important points we discussed during our time together. Encouraging your patients and their loved ones to fully understand their disease and treatment plans includes having the highlights of the plan and instructions written down, giving patient literature, and useful websites for further education. This increases the likelihood of your patient taking action for a healthier outcome.

Patients do not always comprehend much of what is said during hospitalizations, nor after procedures where they have been sedated. During these times, they are under a lot of emotional and physical stress. I often find that they will only hear one or two key phrases and that is it. Like "There's nothing we can do." If it's during a stressful situation in which they need education, it is always important to write out instructions, plan on reeducating at the next visit, and back up your education with patient literature as we spoke about before. Try not to overwhelm them with too much at one time, try small amounts of information at a time. Continue to check in with them to see what their level of understanding is and give them an opportunity to ask questions frequently.

When you are making any medication changes, make sure to be clear on what you want the patient to be on and what you want the patient to stop. On many occasions, I have not communicated well with this point, believing I was clear as day when speaking with my patients, and thinking they understood that I wanted them to stop one medication and take another. In reality, they would continue the old medications, adding the one I ordered to it because I was not clear in stating that they needed to stop the old medicine. We are not always on the same page. What makes perfect sense to us has no bearing with our patients sometimes. I always have a full medication list printed and will write instructions to the side to either continue, stop, or increase beside each drug. If I add anything, it will be on the list with the instructions. Yes, it is tedious, but I want the patient to understand and comply fully with my plan for them. In my experience, this is probably the most important thing I may do for my patients.

If I order any testing or procedures, I write that on a note as well for the patient and I tell them the order of importance. If you are sending the patient to the cardiologist and you are ordering an echocardiogram too, don't you think it would be nice if the patient had that first before visiting the cardiologist. The patient needs to know, do not schedule the cardiologist visit before the echocardiogram is completed. You may know that it goes without saying, because medically, it makes perfect sense to you, but we have to realize, not all of our patients have the insight and understanding that we do.

Take the time, write down your plan of action in the order you want accomplished. This will save everyone, especially your patients, headaches and multiple nonproductive visits. If you are lucky enough to have staff members that can do this for you, take advantage and delegate this task to them. I can tell you that I have recently left the dermatologist's office and he gave me three types of ointments and creams for my face. He never told me what order I needed to put these on, so I had to call and ask which one goes first. These types of instructions are not on the prescription label, but they will make a difference in results.

Be Confident

When I worked in my very first job it was in GI, I would often do paracenteses on a regular basis. However, when I first started performing them I was scared, and can remember being in my office getting sweaty and nervous before I would walk back to the procedure room. I knew how to do them, and I was great at them, but I was still concerned of all the complications that could occur. I knew my patients certainly did not want to see some timid 24-year-old with shaky hands and a look of terror coming back to do their procedure, so I had to make a decision to gear-up, put on a confident smile and walk back and get the procedure done and take care of them the best way that I could. It really was just a simple attitude adjustment.

Patients need to see that you present yourself in a confident manner. It seems to me that they have much more confidence in treatment recommendations when I present my recommendations in a confident way. Learn to present yourself this way. You are great at what you do. You are not an imposter. You have trained diligently to right where you are. Be confident in what you know and be confident in your skills.

"Hey Nurse"

You can't have a book about being a PA without addressing the issue that some of your patients will call you a nurse or ask if you are one. Every PA that I know has been asked this question over and over again. I am still called "*nurse*" by new patients to our practice all the time. I'm also asked when I'll finish school and finally become a doctor. That might sound offensive to you in the beginning, but eventually, you will get used to it. I strongly believe that it is the patient's way of getting to know you a little bit better.

See these questions as an opportunity to educate them on PAs if they have not had experience with our profession. Answer their questions kindly and politely. I will often relay how many years I have already been through and that I am happy where I am. Sometimes I add that as a PA, I spend more time visiting with patients than I ever would have if I were a physician.

There are so many things to be concerned with, don't waste your time being offended by patients asking if you are a nurse or when you are going to complete your training.

I have just as many patients call me doctor as I do nurse. When I correct them, many respond with, "Well, you may not be a doctor, but you are my doctor!" To that, I usually respond, "Call me Rachel, please."

It's all about finding the balance to give a professional and appropriate reply. Even though we have come a long way from where we used to be, our profession can be confusing to patients. As PAs are becoming more and more established, and as we all get more involved in PA organizations and much needed legislation, these issues will definitely diminish.

Issues, We All Got Them

Patients will tell you the most intimate details of their lives, and I have to say, at times, it can be overwhelming. I have heard of patient's past stories of sexual abuse, violent and traumatic deaths of children and spouses, violent crimes, and the most horrible financial difficulties you can imagine.

One of my patients told me how he got into an argument with a co-worker at his home. At some point, the argument turned violent, and the co-worker stabbed him and left him to die. Not only did he stab him, but before he left, he set the patient's house on fire. The patient had some of the worst burn scars I have ever seen. When I asked him about how he dealt with his anger toward the person, he told me, "You know, Rachel, he actually saved my life. Had he not set my house on fire, I would have bled to death. But because of the smoke coming from the house, someone called 911, and I was saved." He was grateful for this complete jerk setting his home on fire. Wow! That was not at all what I would expect. Others in his place would be so angry and resentful. It was a lesson of forgiveness at its best. That day, I realized that if he can forgive someone like that, I should be able to forgive anyone who has wronged me and find the good in every situation.

The pain and tragedies that you are told can genuinely be difficult to deal with. This is why I have chosen to listen to their stories, encourage them in any way I can, learn from their mistakes, and be thankful for my life. Someone always has it worse. I encourage you to listen, learn, and then leave it at work. Do yourself a favor, and do not take your patient's issues home with you. If you are like many, you have enough problems of your own, so you don't need anyone else's.

If you find it difficult to leave things at work, go back to the chapter about taking care of yourself. If you are in a specialty where the nature of what you deal with each day weighs you down and becomes too much of a burden for you, consider changing jobs.

You have to protect yourself and your time away from work. It is essential to your well-being to take a mental and sometimes physical break from work to home. Come up with a routine to transition from work to home. Wash your hands, meditate, or exercise as soon as you get home. Some people do something either physically or visually to end their day. That might be waiting until the last thing they do is take off their jacket to make the transition out of work. They might also envision putting down a piece of baggage at the back door to signal to themselves they are in "home" mode now. They will hit a gong or clap their hands. Having this type of signal may help you with leaving work stress at work. What signal will work for you?

I have laughed and cried with patients. It is truly an honor that they want to share their lives with me. Take this vulnerability they share as an opportunity to encourage them to do better for themselves and think better of themselves. So many people have not been encouraged to truly live and enjoy their lives. They do not realize they are steering their own ship. Each and every day, you get many opportunities to be a positive encouragement to them. If you got into medicine to make a positive impact and change people's lives for the better, this is your chance.

Each patient is your platform for positive change!

Bring It In For A Landing

Have you ever had a patient that keeps repeating the same thing over and over again? Have you ever wondered, "Did she just tell me for the fourth time about her chest pain she had twenty-five years ago?" And things like, "Oh my Lord, when are you ever going to shut up?" Patients can be wordy in their conversations, and sometimes they don't stay on track at all. Although you need to be respectful and not interrupt, there are times when you need to get back on track and redirect them as best you can. This redirection is truly an art of finding what works best for you. A couple of phrases I use are:

"I want to go back to the pain that you were describing just a minute ago. Let's explore this more."

"Ok, let's get back to the shortness of breath that you came in to talk with me about today."

"I hear that you're having aches and pains in your knees, but you came to cardiology today about the stress test results for your chest pain. Let's talk about this first."

You have to realize that you may be the only person they will interact with on the day they see you. Some people live alone and have no one to talk to all day. They look forward to coming and visit with you. Their visit with you is their only social outlet. I have learned to say after indulging in some fun conversations, "I could talk all day about the stock market, but I guess I better get moving or I'm going to have patients getting upset that I'm not running on time."

I know of a physician that, when he is done with his appointment, and the patient continues to talk about irrelevant things, he moves for a handshake with his patient, adding with a kind voice, "Tell me bye now!" I'm not sure that this is the best way. I haven't used it, but I totally get it why he would do it this way. We have to be timely with our appointments and mindful of the other patients waiting. There is undoubtedly an art to this redirection of the patient that you will figure out along your way.

Keeping It Professional

Several years ago, one of my close friends, who was a provider, was murdered in her home by a patient's wife. The wife suspected my friend was having an affair with her husband. I could not believe it. She was a kind and thoughtful physician and always had an ethical perspective. The news of her murder was devastating. I'm not sure of any of the truth to the stories. I have absolutely no details. All I heard were rumors. Did she really get involved with one of her patients? Was any of what we heard on the news true? What was going on? How could it come to this?

Do not cross any boundaries with patients ever. I don't know how to express this enough. Protect yourself, protect your loved ones, and protect your patients. Whatever it is, it will not be worth it. Not that I am all that, but I have been asked out for dinner and drinks more times than I care to admit by both patients and their family members. I haven't been even remotely interested, but I was polite in saying no and changing the subject quickly or getting them out the door. Say *no*, be firm, and redirect the conversation. If they continue to pursue you, continue to be firm, say that you are in a relationship, or whatever you need to. Please do not get yourself into any trouble. And never leave this issue open-ended. Don't let them ask you, "So, you're sayin' there's a chance?"

Our patients are our business. They are the reason to get up in the morning and they keep us gainfully employed. We are here to serve, respect, and treat them with dignity. You have a platform every day to do your best and be your best and encourage your patients in the same way. How you treat them by listening to them, being patient with them, and educating them is of utmost importance and what they deserve to get healthy and live their best life.

Chapter 6

Helpful Tips for Working Well With Staff Members

None of us, including me, ever do great things. But we can all do small things, with great love, and together we can do something wonderful.

—Mother Teresa

As a PA, you have the opportunity to work with so many different types of people from multiple different backgrounds. Whether you work in a solo physician practice or a large medical center area, you will work with, either via phone, email, or in person, numerous medical personnel. It is essential to do your best to be kind, courteous, and professional with all of these people. Every single person has an important role and is valuable in some way. It is your job to work together to create a cohesive team so you can treat your patients with the type of care they deserve. You are a leader. Make it your priority to show excellence in your behavior toward the people you work with. Remind yourself that just because you are in leadership and sometimes authoritarian position, you are no better than the other people you work with. And of course, always be respectful. Always take the higher road.

How You Doin'?

Have you walked a mile in some of your staff member's shoes yet? Do you know what they do for your practice or hospital each and every day? Learn what the people you work with do and how they do it. If you get a good understanding of their position, struggles, and value they add to your team, you can become more successful at your own job. Check in with them, see how they are doing, and ask if they need anything to be more effective in their position. When people feel valued for the work they are doing, they will want to continue to perform in excellent ways.

Take time to learn the different aspects of the practice or hospital you are working in. For example, while working in cardiology, I primarily worked in the outpatient setting. However, when I had time, I spent time in the cath lab, echocardiography lab, and I also spent time with the coders and billers. When you take time to learn the ins-and-outs of the practice and hospital, it gives you a clearer understanding of the issues that each department has and what you can do to help make them be more successful. You may learn that you need to educate your patients more effectively on what they can expect when they go to the common procedures that you order, or who in billing is the right person to speak with. Be open to learning and helping those around you to be more efficient in their own positions.

Kindness

I also feel that when I have taken time to get to know and show appreciation for the people I work with, they are more likely to help me out when I need it most and sometimes with a better attitude. This especially applies to those that I frequently ask to do things for me, like working a patient in or calling a patient back for me or faxing something for me.

Do not issue any demands. Kindly and respectfully ask and **always say thank you**. Just like you want to hear appreciation from the physicians that you work with, your staff wants to hear that you appreciate them as well. Tell them, show them, and be respectful. Take them to lunch every once in a while, bring in breakfast or small trinkets of appreciation. Celebrate their accomplishments with them. This may seem silly, but it will help boost morale and create a positive working environment. I even like writing small note cards or emails of appreciation to the staff and also to their managers. Keep a box of thank you cards in your desk. It won't take that much time to jot a little thank you note down and leave it on their desk.

Encourage your staff members to further their career, and continue to strive for excellence. You may be the only person in their life that encourages them. Each of us has enough stressors at home. I am sure they could use some guidance and affirmation. When you see that your staff needs help or additional resources, you may want to go out of your way to help them get what they need. You might be the only one who observes that they are overworked and need additional help with clinic, scheduling or even some new equipment. Speak up for them.

One of my favorite people I worked with in the VA system was one of the environmental engineers. He was always so lovely and kind and would take care of anything that I asked of him. We frequently sat down for a few minutes on Friday afternoons after I got done with my clinic to visit and catch up for the week. We talked about football; he is a Steelers fan and I am a Chiefs fan, baseball, politics and relationships. You name it; we talked about it over those seven years of Fridays.

You never know who you will befriend. Keep an open mind and applaud those around you that do something right. I promise you that they need your encouragement too.

Explain Yourself

I strongly believe in the "why" of doing things. I try to educate the staff around me on disease processes, treatments, and procedures, so they have a clear understanding of what we are treating, what it is we are doing, and why it is crucial to get things done in a timely and step-by-step specific manner. When they understand the why behind what you are trying to accomplish, they are more likely to be on board with your process. They can also help your process work more efficiently by proposing even better ideas. Be open to their input.

Share your knowledge and educate your staff so that you are all on the same page. Take time to have a lunch-and-learn with the team you work closely with. Explain the basics of pathophysiology and treatment plans for the different common diseases you see in the office. Describe the importance of the routine laboratory tests you are ordering and how they help you in your clinical decision making. Tell them about the procedures and surgeries that your patients may have and the risks associated with them. Taking time to educate those that you work with will not only help them understand the nature of your practice, but it will also help you gain respect amongst your office staff as an expert in the field. It might help your physicians who may have thought of doing something like that, but just never took the time to get it done.

That's What She Said

In medicine as well as in any other field, there is always office drama to be found somewhere—if not everywhere. I would advise you to distance yourself as much as possible from it. Strive to have the reputation that when people come to you about their problems, whether work or home-related, you keep it between yourselves. Be encouraging, but do not get involved with the office/hospital drama. It only makes you look poorly. Plus, if you keep things to yourself, you will have a good reputation amongst the people that you work with, and you will likely have a better idea of what is going on so that you can help to facilitate change for the better when the opportunity arises.

Even in a large city, word gets around about the quality and the character of individuals, reputation of offices, and the physicians' expertise. Many times, employees, including PAs, doctors, nurses, and medical staff, having experience within a particular specialty, will go to a different practice within that same specialty down the street or across town. Their knowledge and opinions of the staff from the practice they came from follow them. So when you look for another position within the same specialty, you can guarantee your future employer will ask anyone who might know you or your reputation, what you are like.

A physician once told me that he knew I was great at my job because he had spoken about my job performance and reputation with a former fellow from the VA I had worked with several years ago. I had not seen that fellow in years and honestly, I did not know that he stayed in the area. I was so happy to hear of this and then scared to death of what all the other fellows had said about me. I hope I was as helpful to them and did not seem too inconvenienced that they would only see two patients in an afternoon during our clinics together. Have you seen this too? Some fellows are somewhat slow to get to the clinic and always the first ones to have a meeting across town.

I have worked with and help train many fellows and medical students coming through the VA system, and likely, if you are in a large institution, you will too. Take time to be kind, helpful, and teach them as much as you can. The education and help you give these fellows, residents, and students allows you a fantastic opportunity to make an even bigger impact for patients down the road.

It always pays to be kind, courteous, respectful, and help those around you be better at their job.

Carry On

Many of you may find that you are in a position, and a nurse practitioner has the same role as you do within your job. I strongly suggest that you don't get involved in the whole nurse practitioner/PA argument. I believe there is a role and place and room for all of us. We all had the opportunity to do our home-work on the two professions before choosing ours. Be the best at what you do, and good things will follow.

You also may find that you are the liaison between staff mem-bers and your physician. Sometimes physicians may have that persona of being intimidating or unapproachable, and you may be inadvertently chosen to be the go-between because you spend the most time with that particular physician and have a good rapport with him or her. Hell, sometimes even other physicians will have you represent their interests to your physician on their behalf. Be respectful and confidential on all parties' behalf and do whatever biddin' you see necessary!

When you work well with your staff and are kind, courteous, informative, respectful, and appreciative, you will find that you will build lifelong friendships, positive morale, and you will all be working on common ground. Building strong relationships with your staff is vital to treating and caring for patients in the best way that they deserve.

Chapter 7

Developing Purposeful Daily Habits and Organizational Tips for Success

Be humble. Be hungry. And always be the hardest worker in the room.

—Dwayne "The Rock" Johnson
Actor

I have to say, working with patients is the absolute best part of being a PA. There is always someone new to meet, a fascinating story, an intriguing problem, or an interesting disease to treat. And as I see it, there is an opportunity behind each door to encourage our patients and their families. Patients are why we are here.

If you got into medicine to make substantial money, you know you are definitely in the wrong business, right? Yes, practicing medicine is tried and true and stable in financially difficult times, but if you are looking to pull in a nice six-figure bonus, you should probably start looking elsewhere or renegotiate your salary or hours. It may not offer the luxuries of the Wall Street guys, but, it definitely pays the bills though!

Caring for patients is the essence of our practice. They can bring us joy in their stories and in their crazy jokes they want to tell. They can bring us heartache in sharing some of the difficulties in their lives. They challenge us to think beyond the typical everyday pathology and make us want to be better and learn more to help them create a more healthy and longer life. Our patients are the reason we strive to practice excellent medicine and enjoy the day-to-day aspects of our jobs!

I am here to tell you, I have made numerous mistakes in things I have said or asked when speaking to patients and their families. It has taken a while to get some good verbiage down in order to get information I want, without coming off as being completely offensive. And I am sure I have insulted patients and family members by asking questions without thoroughly thinking them through.

I have also been, at times, completely unorganized and inefficient in practice, but, I eventually found success in how I have organized my daily practice within the office and hospital. Being purpose-driven as a PA takes working hard at the little things every day, so you can become more efficient and valuable to your patients and your practice. I want to share with you several pointers I have learned over my career that have helped me become the best version of myself. These ideas help me stay organized and focused, keeping patients at the forefront of what I do. Some things I've picked up along the way from those I have had the privilege to work with, and some I have derived through my inefficiencies.

Marie Kondo-ing Your Day

As a PA, you will face challenges every single day. There is so much to keep up with, and sometimes these challenges can be a bit overwhelming. As we mentioned in Chapter 1, remember every day why you got into medicine and why you do what you do. Let your why motivate you daily.

I don't know if you have heard of Marie Kondo and the Kon-Mari method, but she is an organizer of home and heart. She is all about minimization, optimization, and urges her followers to create an environment around them that sparks joy. How easy is this in our offices? Ugh, it's not. Over my twenty-something years in medicine and traveling around for my latest role as a technical sales specialist, I have been in hundreds—if not thousands of offices. I seriously cannot think of one that seemed like it was well organized or decluttered. I don't know about you, but I just feel better and can be so much more effective if the environment around me is as clean and organized as possible. Sometimes, it's just my way to procrastinate in getting some work done but overall, I know it helps me be more successful when everything is in order around me.

During COVID 19 chaos, as I like to call it, I was able to get my office and home sparkling clean and organized. It was the first time in my life that I knew where every item I owned was located. It was a ton of work. It was dusty, It was dirty, and I had no idea how embarrassingly unorganized I was. I discovered a huge stack of paperwork from my first PA job back in 1996, and I won't even mention the issue of patient privacy that was lost within this mess (for legal purposes, it was immediately shredded.) Once I put in the hours of work and effort and got organized, it was the most freeing feeling in the world. For those of you who like budgets and the freeing feeling a budget can bring, this is for you too!

If you are lucky enough to have an office or a regular area that you sit in, take the time to get your environment around you to the point that it is easy and comfortable to work in. Consider bringing in a couple of lamps instead of using the harsh overhead lighting. Not the ones that are ready to be donated to the thrift store. Go to Marshall's or TJ Maxx and spend less than $100 dollars and get some inexpensive, but nice items that you like. Get some pretty bins that you like to look at to store your paperwork in. Bring in art that speaks to you. If you can't put a nail in the wall, use the 3M command picture hanging strips.

They are so cool. Use pens and notepads that are nice. I am a lover of TUL pens. Don't wait for your office administrator to get things for you, spend some money and invest in items that you like and make you feel great about being there. I know not all PAs have a work area where they can change much, but if you can, it will help to tidy up your surroundings to make your work area more warm and inviting. You spend a lot of time at work; it may as well be in enjoyable surroundings.

Places To Go And People To See

Time and task management is essential to getting home at a decent hour and getting the most done for your patients. Find a way that is best for you to be organized. Make a list and prioritize it. Ask yourself, what are the top items I need to do today that cannot wait until tomorrow? Get these done and move on to the next. Put reminders on your phone calendar to check up on specific tasks you may forget about. I know you want to ignore the paperwork you have to fill out for your patients and the insurance companies, but come up with a plan to get this work done. I always hate tasks hanging over my head, but save some time at the beginning or end of each day to get these types of items accomplished.

You may try batching your work as you go. It's the same mindset of paying bills. Do you pay just one bill at a time? Most people, including myself, wait and pay several bills at one time. There is so much research out there that says batching work leads to better efficiency. I know you are seeing patients and trying to get tasks accomplished in between, but if you do all your emails at once and then move to all of your lab review at once and then all of your calls at once to get them knocked out, this batching may help you save a little time towards the end of the day. If you are completing paperwork for one patient and you have four other paperwork type items that are similar, you will be more productive by getting all of the items done at once while you are in the same mindset of doing paperwork.

The Waiting Game

When I was interviewing for my first job out of PA school, it was with an OB/GYN that I adored. He offered me the position, but I wanted the gastroenterology position that I ended up taking. He was kind, caring, and I could just tell that he was fantastic at his job. While I was waiting for my interview, I could see that his patients were crazy about him. So when I was pregnant with my first child, I chose him as my OB. He was always running late. Ok, when I say late, think up to three hours behind.

He had a busy solo practice, and I really do not know how he managed. He needed a PA, okay, maybe he needed three PAs. However, his office staff was always so kind and polite and kept the waiting room informed of his estimated time of arrival. Three hours is a long time when you are competing with others for the bathroom, but when he came in the door to see me, any irritation from waiting was automatically gone. He had that kind of effect. He even made me feel completely comfortable telling him about peeing myself just about anytime I changed positions. He always sat down, listened to me intently, and gave me the time I needed. He was so worth waiting for that I went back when I was pregnant with my second child as well.

There are several lessons in this story. First, when you are running behind, let your patients know. Either you should stick your head in real quick and let your patients know that you are running late, or you should have someone on your staff notify your patients. Acknowledging your delay shows respect. Patients will be more patient and willing to wait for you if they just understand what is going on. If appropriate, have healthy snack and drink options. If you have materials or magazines for your patients to read while they wait, make sure they are from the current decade. Seriously! Have something available to keep make the wait more tolerable. I know most people are on their phone all of the time, but consider this time as captured attention to educate them on conditions you regularly treat in your office with having brochures available or educational health TV that so many practices are utilizing these days. It would also be a great time to have your patients do surveys that you might need for research purposes.

Next, I love that Dr. Balat always sat down and spoke with me. He gave me his undivided attention. I felt like he was listening and hearing what I had to say. Have you ever had those providers that stand at the door with their hand on the doorknob when they speak to you? How well heard do you feel? How disrespectful can we be as providers? We have to make our patients feel like they are our only concern when we are with them. Please sit down and listen to your patients. They need to feel important, and we must be respectful to them and their time.

Lastly, having an enjoyable waiting area and exam rooms will allow your patients to feel more comfortable in what can already be a very stressful situation. One of the orthopedic surgeons I worked with while I was at Medtronic had a waiting room and patient rooms that were straight out of the 1970s. There was the dark wood paneling, green carpet, grandma's kitchen chairs, flickering fluorescent overhead lighting that swayed back and forth. I did not see a lava lamp, but it would have been a perfect place to have a 70's birthday party. It felt damp and old and musty and gross. Who knows when the carpet had ever been cleaned or the paneling dusted? I know you may not have much control over the decor or vibe of the office, but if you do or if you have your office manager's ear, can you please address this issue for your patient's sake?

Allow Me To Introduce Myself

I know it may be silly that I am telling you to introduce yourself, but you would be surprised at how many providers I have met that fail to introduce themselves or even give a greeting while walking down the hallway. How rude and arrogant are we that we assume everyone knows who we are? And why would we think our patients and staff don't deserve a greeting of hello? I know we are busy but are we too busy for introductions and greetings?

Let me tell you about something that happened only last week when I took my son to a new doctor. Neither he nor his staff introduced themselves to us. New patients do not always know who you are or what role you have. Representatives that are new to your practice have not been stalking your Facebook account to see who you are. Don't let yourself get too busy, with the tasks at hand and the stressors of your day, to introduce yourself.

I always introduce myself to my patients as a PA. This has been one of my spiels. "Hello, my name is Rachel, and I'm the physician assistant who works with Dr. Wolter and Dr. Meredith, our neurosurgeons." If they don't know what a PA is, this is my opportunity to sell the great things PAs can do for them! Surely by now, everyone knows what PAs do? Okay, we are still working on this issue, but we have come a long way from where we were twenty years ago.

Work The Room

As you are introducing yourself, make sure you address all those in the room with the patient. Do you go to a party and just address the host when you walk in? No, you work the room and say hello to everyone. You smile, you greet them, and you introduce yourself. It should be no different with your patients.

Several years ago, when I was dating my husband, we hosted a graduation party for my son. Several of my son's friend's parents attended, and several of my children's dads' friends came. One of the attendees –that I had met a couple of times, but I obviously did not know well—met Jonathan and asked him how the construction business was going. He started laughing and said, "No, I'm Jonathan, 2.0." I had previously dated a guy named John, and my husband's name is Jonathan. Jonathan is not in construction, but the old John was. She was horrified after asking this, but Jonathan played it off so well. He is way beyond being offended by something like this. I had been through a couple of guys. How could she possibly keep up with the Johns and Jonathan in my life?

We all make assumptions. It is part of who we are. We are always trying to put the pieces together. But I am telling you from experience and embarrassment, you just never know who is in the room with your patients. In this day and age of Botox® and JUVÉDERM® and who knows what, I never know if it's the patient's daughter, wife, or mother who is with them. I have simply learned to ask, "And who is this with you today?" instead of being horrified when the patient says, "No, this is not my mother, this is my wife!" or "this is my son, not my grandson!" Have you made this mistake yet, or am I the only one? Why they come back and see me after I have offended them and their family, I do not know!

It can be interesting to see who shows up for your patients in times of illness. Several years ago, I walked into one of my patient's hospital rooms, and he had several ladies by his bedside. He went on to say he was happy to see me and then said, "I'm so glad you came in just now, I wanted to introduce you to my family. This is my wife, Sheila, and this is my girlfriend, Stacey." Then he sat back and laughed at my bewildered expression, and everyone in the room started laughing. As it turned out, they really were his ex-wife and his current girlfriend. I guess that's how it works in their family. At least some folks can still get along! I love it!

More power to them!

Check The Chart

In my first year of medical practice, I worked for a large HMO in Houston. I spent four days a week in gastroenterology, and the other day, I worked at an outlying clinic working in family practice. One day at the family practice office, I was about to go in with one of my patients who had just learned that she was pregnant and was coming in with some concerns before going to the OB/GYN. As I was looking over her chart prior to meeting her for the first time, I noticed that her weight had dropped about 100 pounds within 12 months. I was thinking, "Wow, that's impressive, I wonder how she did that when I can't even lose 5 pounds in a month (and this is in the days before lap band® mind you)."

While I was talking to her, she introduced me to one of her girlfriends whom she had brought along for support. Continuing our conversation, I went about asking her how she lost all the weight. I kept giving her encouragement and praise, but in doing so, I noticed her answers were extremely off and a bit suspicious. In speaking with her, she had come to the clinic that day asking for a same day abortion. Now I don't know about your program, but doing abortions was not part of the *See One, Do One, Teach One* model at our PA school. So I go outside and wait for my attending to ask what to do in this situation. I had not encountered an opportunity for learning like this before and as I was sitting there and sitting there. You know how it is when you are waiting for your attending to walk out and help you and you are looking through the patient chart and contemplating all their strange answers, trying to make sense of it all. Finally, it donned on me. This girl is totally not who she says she is. I don't think she has ever been overweight. Oddly enough, her friend she has with her is overweight. She is using someone else's insurance. Is it her friend's insurance? The friend who is in the room with her? I think it is her friend's. I know it's her friends!

Sure enough, she was using her friend's insurance card. I could not believe it. They were trying to pull a fast one over on me and I caught on. I thought I was the best investigative PA in the whole world at the moment. I needed an award or something for sure! It was drama that eventually involved the practice administrators, and the police. It was a little crazy to say the least. And you know there was no reward. Right?

If a patient history is not adding up, there is a reason. In our economy with fraud and insurance abuse galore, you may even have a little more drama on your hands than you bargained for. Keep digging and keep investigating. I guess that's one good reason to have the patient's picture taken and attached to our EMRs now. I completely believe these pictures help in remembering the patients and their particular case.

All this to say, take time to thoroughly evaluate your patients' medical records before walking in the room. No patient wants to remind you of what you ordered last time they were in. Review your last note if you have seen them before. Do they have any labs or imaging that need to be reviewed beforehand? Know what kind of problem list the patient may have and why they are coming in. Don't just trust the brief info that the medical assistant gives you. Thoroughly go through the consult and supporting documents available. Review their medications. This information will at least steer you in the right direction to get things started off well and help you appear well-organized.

When I would get my clinic list the day before or the morning of, I would take some time to go through each patient that was coming in for the day and jot some notes down. If they had imaging or labs or results that needed to be reviewed I would take a look at it and then if I needed one of the physicians to look at it as well, I would try to review this information with them first and have a rough plan before the patient ever got to clinic.

If you take time to review this information up front, then this will save you and the patient some wait time in the future.

Say What?

Ok, so one afternoon, I'm seeing a new patient, who is with his wife, in the clinic and going through his past surgical history and for some reason, please do not ask me why, but after he tells me he had a vasectomy I ask him "And who did that for you?" Why? Oh, why did I even ask this question? I don't know any vasectomy doctors; I'm not in the search for one, although I certainly don't want any more kids in the mix. But, all things considered, I was thinking, "What physician or what hospital or year did that surgical procedure take place in?" Again, not that I needed to know, good gravy-he was probably in his 70s or so!

So, without skipping a beat, he says, "My neighbor."

And then I ask with full curiosity, "What hospital does he or she work at?"

And he says in his best drawl, "No, he doesn't work at a hospital. He works down at the Ford Plant."

Hold up. What did he just say? Despite all my efforts, this is the end of my straight face. Did he just say the Ford Plant? The Ford Plant as in Ford trucks and cars? He did mean the Ford Plant. The patient's new wife and I started laughing hysterically at how ridiculous all of this sounded.

The patient continued, "Well, he was a medic back in the military!"

And my teasing response, "I had no idea performing vasectomies were part of a combat medic's training, but that's interesting." I'm not sure that I ever felt comfortable or even understood what had happened with my patient, and frankly, it didn't matter, but it has to be one of the funniest surgical history interviews ever.

Getting a proper history of present illness and past medical history is one of the most entertaining aspects of being in healthcare. I enjoy learning about my patients and who I am working with. You can learn so much by asking such few questions about people. I have learned about exciting travels, jobs, marriages, deaths, vasectomies. And the list goes on.

This is definitely where the art of keeping a straight face comes into play, and the tendency to harshly judge needs to be thrown out the window. In your practice, you will deal with patients who are cousins who are married to each other, murderers, thieves, convicts, child-molesters, and rapists. You will also work with patients who are teachers, pastors, survivors, and givers! And sometimes you will never know the difference. Be kind, be thoughtful, and be forgiving and give exceptional care regardless.

Getting a thorough history is what will make you shine as a PA. Many times, your patients will tell you everything you need to know about what is going on with them. It is your job to interrupt as little as possible and to redirect and really focus on what is at hand. I know I mentioned this previously, but it is essential to get their story straight. I often ask patients, "Okay, so this is what I am hearing,…" and then I retell the key aspects of what I have heard and then ask, "Is this correct?" and sometimes I get it right and sometimes they need to retell some aspects of what is going on. This is where I didn't realize I was going to be an investigative reporter. But we are. We are to relate in our documentation the who, what, when, where, and why. We must accurately, specifically, and succinctly retell our patient's stories as we document.

Let's Get Physical

As a student, you will practice every minute detail of the physical exam. It is imperative that you learn the importance of what every normal and abnormal finding is. Just the other day, I was trying to figure out what kind of hearing loss I was experiencing and thinking to myself, "Ok, if the Weber test lateralizes to the left ear and that is the ear I am having the problem with, what does that mean?" Ugh! How easily we forget! So, years later, I went back to the physical exam book I have had since training to look it up! I keep it nearby as I reference it regularly. Keep ahold of your physical exam book and references. They definitely come in handy when changing specialties.

Now that you know how to do the physical exam and all the parts of it, how judgy are you when you have to visit your provider and they do an exam on you? I have to say, I am very blessed to be healthy and well and have had to be evaluated rarely. But, when I have had any type of physical exam, even by providers with good reputations, it has been a shoddy job. I mean, why bother? If you don't do a thorough physical exam, you are doing a disservice to your patients. Don't just go through the motions of doing the physical exam to make the patient think they are getting their money's worth out of you. Take your time, expose the skin, look, listen, palpate.

I can tell you I have had patients come in and tell me their providers don't evaluate them the way I do. And, I promise I did not make up any new cool physical exam techniques. I perform a standard methodical appropriate physical exam. Take your time. When you do a proper exam enough times, you will be aware of when something abnormal comes along. This helped me tremendously with murmurs. I had heard enough normal that I can pick up abnormal super-fast! Always practice proper technique as well. Do right for your patients. You examine patients all the time. They deserve the best care you can give them. They may only experience or receive your care once. Give them your best.

Several years ago, we had a patient who was quite elderly come in. He was telling us about how he was doing, and we were asking him about his pacemaker. It had been a while since he was seen at our facility, and we were asking him where he was following up for his device checks. He was charming, but a bit confused. He told us how he didn't remember having a pacemaker but wanted us to take a look at his pocket watch that he had been having problems setting the time. Later during the physical exam, when we went to look at the device site, the pacemaker battery was entirely outside of the skin, with the leads still attached. His 'pocket watch' was his pacemaker, a classic Twiddler's Syndrome. And the device/pocket watch was perfectly shiny, with the manufacturer name clear as day!

There is no telling how long that pacemaker had been dangling on the outside of his chest. It had to have been a long time; there was no open wound or crusty scab. Nothing. Who else had he seen that never exposed the skin to take a look at what was going on? He certainly had some other issues, but luckily and surprisingly, he did not have an infection. He deserved better care and a proper exam each time he was seen. And, I won't even tell you about his toenails. That's just a different 'long' story altogether. Always inspect the areas you are examining. You just never know when you might find an eroded device, a strange scar, or a fun tattoo with a special meaning your patient is willing to share.

Ok, since you asked, or I just really want to tell; I did have a patient who told me he won many a bet over one of his tattoos. He would bet them his cock (his word) was lower down his leg than theirs. There was a tattoo of a rooster on the inside of his leg near his ankle. I swear it! He said people loved it so much that they didn't mind handing over their money to him at all. Of course, there is a penis joke in this book and a story about comparing them. And yes, I made him show me. His tattoo, that is. INSPECTION complete!

Smooth Operator

Surgery and procedure days seem to be forever long and crazy hectic. It seems I would only remember things that I needed to get done once I got into the OR and was three layers deep in lead and gloves and scrub bottoms that liked to come untied. I would have to try to remember everything for six to twelve hours later when and all I could think about was getting to the bathroom as fast as possible, or I would have to kindly ask the staff to call the office and have someone else help me out. I had to find ways to keep on task and keep it together before, during, and after these days.

Always check in with the family before and after procedures when possible. I find that many PAs are the one person families can truly count on when their loved ones are in the hospital or having procedures or surgery. We are the ones who take the time, listen, explain, and educate. They are anxious about their loved ones and need to have as much information as possible. Take time with them to help them through this as well. They are the ones who will remember your instructions and help implement them.

Set expectations, educate appropriately, be thoughtful, and stay until their questions are complete. Check in with them to make sure they understand what you are saying. Have them repeat to you what they just heard; this can be a doozy, and you may sometimes wonder why you checked in to see if they understood. I cannot tell you how many times I have had to repeat myself. I swear I don't speak another language well. I know I said it clearly. They just got stuck on one word I said, and their brain did not allow for them to make it past that one word. Who knows what that one word can be for them to get stuck on. Was it a four-week recovery? Was it no work for eight weeks? Was it Percocet? Was it a catheter? Was it no sexual intercourse? Regardless, having them repeat instructions to you with clarity is vital for you to have fewer calls in the middle of the night, better compliance, and a faster recovery.

It had been fifteen years since I had been in the OR as a student when I went moved over to neurosurgery. I was so nervous and a bit timid at the beginning. I had to choose to quickly overcome my fear and speak with confidence during surgery. When our patients are on the table and cannot speak for themselves, we must always be on the lookout for them. The longer they are under anesthesia, the more likely they are to have problems. We must be efficient at this time as best as possible. It is of the utmost importance to be aware and alert during procedures, traumas, and surgeries.

Pay attention, learn quickly, and ask for clarification when needed. Patient safety is always a top priority, so it is essential to always be aware of your surroundings. A wise piece of advice one of my physicians said to me is, "It is imperative to be the calm in the storm." While everyone is panicking and wondering what to do, realize that you are the provider and you are there to reassure good medical decision-making. You are the one everyone else is looking to. If you panic, chaos will ensue. If you remain calm and collected, your staff will follow suit.

Be the eyes and ears for your surgeon when they need you. Always be thinking about the patient. Ask questions sparingly. Protect the sterile field. Check the monitors. Be bold when required, and speak up clearly on behalf of your patient. Always anticipate the next moves for your doctors so that the staff can have items ready before being asked. Lead wisely and with gratefulness to everyone in the room you are working with.

A little soapbox moment—help the staff you are working with. You are not too good to help bring the patient back to the room or out of the room. You are not too good to help position the patient correctly and get the patient set up. Help ensure everything is set up well so you can be effective and be able to anticipate needs that may arise. Everyone you work with deserves for you to show up as a team player in all aspects of your job. And, back to the book.

Write That Down

Documentation is vital in our profession. It is critical to document fully the proper history, findings, and recommendations that you give patients and their families. Thorough documentation can save you from an orange jumpsuit. In my first position at an HMO, which is no longer in business, I dictated all of my notes. One day I received a call from one of our administrators asking me to stop dictating so much information because it cost too much money. I was so nice and apologetic and willingly agreed to be wise and succinct with my words. I promptly got off the phone turned around and continued dictating in the way I knew best....with all the words and information I thought necessary to put in the chart.

Several years later, that same practice was named in a lawsuit. I, along with the other numerous providers the patient had seen over several years were all named in it. Talk about anxiety, worry, embarrassment, and total freak out! It was a nightmare! I got served papers at my house with my brand new baby on my hip!

Guess what? It was my detailed documentation that released me from any wrongdoing in that case. It has been my only case thus far that I have been named in, and later dropped from, but one trip to the attorney's office to give a deposition and you will be thanking your lucky stars that you documented all important aspects of your encounter with the patient. You will never be sorry that you took the time to document properly and thoroughly.

I have messed up on documenting as well, more times than I even care to admit. I have had several occasions come back, and I have thought to myself, "I should have documented what I said to that patient on the phone." Whether it is that you offered to see the patient in the office ahead of their scheduled appointment or that they called to tell you about their chest pain, and you recommended that they go to the ER. Always take time to cover your bases with detailed documentation. I promise you, it's worth your time and sleep at night. And if someone complains that your dictation is costing too much, ask them if they are willing to cover your legal fees and go to prison for your lack of details.

Code Words

Speaking of proper documentation, I wanted to address something with you that I think some of our training has failed to teach in the past years, and that is proper coding of your encounters with your patients. Maybe things are better and more precise, my goodness it has been a while since I have been in school, but even in practice, I feel a little inadequate at this. Is it just me, or do you feel that way too?

Coding is how you and I make our money and make our practice money and keep our jobs. If you have proper training and code correctly, it can make the difference in hundreds of thousands of dollars for your practice. And if you improperly code, it can mean a large fine from insurance companies and Medicare. We must get this right!

I recommend you to take all the coding classes your practice will allow. And if your practice has not hired a PA before, it would be wise for you to become adept in knowledge of proper coding for your practice. In addition, it would be wise to always know how much you are billing for every encounter, every procedure, and every surgery that you complete. This is how you justify your position, attain raises, and keep track of bonuses and productivity. You should know how much insurance reimburses PAs in every situation you are involved in. It is well worth the investment for you to even attend these coding classes on your own time and dime to learn proper techniques that may save your practice money or may be able to bill at a larger level based on your performance.

In every practice I have been in, I make a point of becoming friends with the people who code for the practice. These coders can help you in keeping track of your productivity and help you know your worth. I have been involved in one surgery alone in which my first assistant fee alone would have covered more than several months of my salary. I always like to know that I am earning my keep. You should too. Invest your time, know your worth, and use it to your advantage.

You certainly may have gotten into medicine to help and encourage your patients and to become a productive member of society, but also remember, you have to make a living. You are there to make your practice money, and you certainly don't want them coming to you saying you are not billing enough to cover your salary. You are charging enough. Be proactive and find out just how much you are bringing in for your practice or hospital. If someone tells you they don't know, do not believe them. Someone will be able to help you find out.

Poker Face

Are you able to keep it together when your patients tell you things that just do not make sense? Having a poker face is one aspect of medicine I continually find myself struggling with. I just happen to be one of those people that when I'm happy, you know it, and when I'm sad or mad, you can just tell. My kids will tell you they can read my face from the rearview mirror. They immediately know they are in trouble or have moved completely over the line of inappropriateness. For the most part, with patients, I can keep it together. However, I have found it sometimes difficult not to burst out in laughter at what patients, and their family members, tell me or bring in to me.

So, be prepared when you work in gastroenterology, and you ask what someone's stool looks like, they may have just taken a picture of it for you with their cell phone, or brought in a frozen sample of it in a butter dish for you to take a gander at! It's true. It happens! I have bitten the sides of my cheeks to where they are raw at times, and I have had to get up and leave the room at some of the worst smells. You will see and hear all kinds of crazy, just like we spoke about before, try to keep it together the best you can for your patients. The last thing you want is for them to feel bad for being honest and vulnerable with you. Sometimes I just move quickly to the next item on my agenda and focus there so that I don't dwell too much on whatever it was that was so distracting.

Testing, Testing 1, 2, 3!

With the rising costs of healthcare, practicing medicine is getting more and more expensive. Unless you are going to do something with the results, why order a test or procedure for a patient? Have you learned to ask yourself this question before ordering procedures and tests? It is wise to ask yourself this question for every test you order. If you are going to continue your plan of care regardless of the results, there is no need to waste a patient's time, your time, your staff's time, or anyone's money. Whatever you order, it should be actionable.

You also need to consider the financial resources that you could be wasting. For example, if a patient comes in with back pain and right leg that has slightly progressed since the last MRI of her lumbar spine, but refuses surgical intervention, why order another MRI? Especially since you are documenting that she refuses to have any surgical intervention?

Sometimes what I do is offer the procedure and allow the patient to decline to have it done. I explain that we can certainly order the test to see what the results are, but if they are still not going to change their mind regardless of the results, then they may not want to waste their time or resources to seek these results. Since I have worked for the government for most of my career, I have to consider that I am spending tax-payer dollars with everything I do. You must also ask if there is something cheaper and as good as the more expensive option before ordering any test. Notice I said as good as. Do not order a sub-par test that has less accuracy, sensitivity, or specificity. Order what is best for the patient. Order what you would want for your loved one. Order the test or procedure that will give the most accurate results. And as always, document what you are doing and what you will use the information for, or document what you are not doing and why.

Please do your patients the favor of following up with them regarding their results. Don't make them sit at home, wondering their results or thinking that no news is good news. I encourage you to commit to yourself to follow up on any bad news or abnormal tests that need an explanation. Your patients want to hear from you. They do not want to hear from one of your staff members unless it's good news. If you have your staff call the patient, they may not be able to answer questions as thoroughly as you. This is where your expertise and guidance is needed. They do not want to hear bad news by reading about it on the patient portal, either.

Your patients deserve to have clear communication from you. They are paying you for your expertise and recommendations. You know exactly how it feels for your provider to give you a call to go over results. You feel like you are a priority to them. You may think that you don't have time to call with results but I encourage you to find the time and take it. This is caring for your patients. If you can't find the time, schedule another appointment with your patients, so you can thoroughly go over their results, giving them time to ask and get answers for all of their questions.

Phone A Friend

We had to call and let one of our patients know that we could no longer refill his narcotic medication because he had a positive urine drug screen for marijuana and cocaine. He called several times, asking for a refill, and the assistant kept telling him it was impossible. After the third time he spoke with her and she let me know about the incident, I called the patient back to let him know the reasons why we would not be refilling his medication. Without skipping a beat replied, "Well, when do I get to reapply?" Reapply? I didn't know it was an application process. I simply repeated that we would not be refilling his medication and that was that. He needed to hear this from me. No more calls.

You will likely get numerous calls a week from your patients. If they are like many patients, they will not want to speak with your assistant, but directly with you. They want to get the information straight from the horse's mouth. And sometimes they won't even tell the staff what it is they want to talk to you about as they want to keep the conversation as private as possible.

Kindly call them back. Be polite and respectful. Take time to educate your patient. If they are a frequent flier caller, if you take time to educate upfront and set boundaries, this may save you and your staff, from more calls in the future. Occasionally patients will want to hold you hostage over the phone and treat this time as a consultation or as their social time because they have no one else to speak with during the day. Answer what you can and then tell them to write down all of their questions, bring them to their next appointment to address them one-by-one.

In addition, try to get to your phone calls and messages during the day as best as you can. If they pile up too much during the day, it can be overwhelming to get through at the end of the day when all you can think about is getting home to Netflix and a glass of wine. And don't forget to document what you spoke about. You will want to make sure they have a clear understanding of the conversation. You can ask, "Can you repeat to me your understanding of what we just spoke about? I want to make sure we are on the same page."

FaceTime / You Need To Represent!

You may not realize it, but as the PA in your practice and specialty, you will often be the glue that holds everything together. You may be more readily available to your patients than the physician or physicians you work with. You may be the one making the everyday decisions that represent your practice. Every time you work with anyone in your practice, hospital, or referring offices, you are the face of your practice. Make sure you speak with respect and know your limitations.

Once referring physicians get to know me, they often call me, rather than the physicians that I work with. I am more easily accessible; more prompt in my return calls, and can get them an answer they are looking for much quicker than them waiting for my doctors to get back with them. By being the face of the practice and being the accessible one, you free up your physician to do what they do best.

When you represent your physician and your practice well, you make everyone look great, including our profession. I can tell you that I have gotten more job offers and referring physicians telling me they need a PA after they work with me. They see the benefits and the easing of duties a PA brings to the table for their practice.

If you are looking for a new job, this is a great way to network and know the practices and physicians you might work with in the future. When you are nice and polite, and you know what you are talking about, then you get more referrals for your practice, you justify your job, and you have more job security. You are making yourself indispensable!

Again, it is crucial in any situation to know your limitations. If you do not know the answer, then tell them you will get the answer and get right back to them. And, by all means, do what you say you are going to do! I promise you will gain more respect when doing this.

If you are in a specialty practice, it is often hard not to criticize the referring physician for making poor medical decisions and sending in bad referrals. We all get, and we all make bad referrals. It happens! Remember, if they knew the answer to the questions they were asking, they would not need to be referring to you, and you would be out of a job. Our job depends on these referrals, whether they are bad or good. Be thankful they don't know the answer, and they need you to help them! Be grateful for the easier consult with a straightforward answer. It is nice to have those types of consults some days. Every day we get to choose the spin we will put on our perspective. Choose a positive one and give the primary care and internists a break, they have to know so much about everything, and it is difficult for them to keep up. Hell, it is difficult for any of us to keep up with all aspects of medicine!

If you are in primary care and you are about to call a specialist to ask a question, please consider asking your attending physician before calling the specialist. This double-checking with your physician first will save you from being the one they are speaking about behind your back. Come on, you and I both know this happens frequently. But still, if you need to call and you can actually get the specialist on the phone, by all means, do so. Seek to get the answers your patients deserve. You are their best advocate!

Never be offended when a physician calls and does not want to speak with you or does not want to have you seeing their patients. Yes, this has happened to me and I both hated it and was completely offended by it. Please realize this has absolutely nothing to do with you, but with their pride. It is hard for some doctors—if not most—to admit that PAs know more than they do in some areas. I promise, once they get to know you and know your reputation, over time, they will come to rely on you just as much as the physician you work with and sometimes even more so, due to your accessibility and knowledge. In our profession, you will continually have to earn respect. With your courtesy and clinical acumen, you will easily accomplish this.

Your patients will also go back and let the referring provider know how they were treated and who treated them. Trust me; your patient will say it like it is, good or bad. Wouldn't you? The saying above by Maya Angelou is so dead on. Patients will always remember how you made them feel. Continue to do what you do best. Continue to care and treat your patients with kindness and respect, and professionalism. It will not go unnoticed or unrewarded.

Vote For Your Local Representative

Many of us have differing views on sales representatives within the office. You will likely deal with many different sales reps during your practice. There are the few pushy, salesy, obnoxious ones, and then there are many more representatives, technical and clinical specialists who can be extremely helpful to you and your practice. The ones I worked with in neurosurgery and cardiology were truly an extension of our practice. They can have some great information about their product and reimbursements that could benefit the way you treat patients and the way you make money for the practice. Think about it, they are expertly trained in their product, and it is their job to know everything about it, the competition, and all the legal and on-label uses. They will likely know way more than do over their product or service. They can be your go-to for new products, medications and more. And, if there is a new product that I am not familiar with and I am still deciding whether to use it, I ask them for the literature to review for myself. They have access to these articles that are sometimes difficult to get your hands on.

Realize they are there to inform you of their company's product. They are a direct advertisement. Do you always get mad when you see a billboard, a commercial, or an Instagram ad? You should not get mad at them for being there to speak with you. They are just an in-person advertisement. These representatives can be quite beneficial to you. For several years, I've had the privilege of working with many reps both as a clinical and technical specialist. I see it from this side and view my role as simply an educator. I educate providers and staff on products, the literature, how the product might be of value to their patients in their practice, when and how to use it, and the cost alternatives. I educate, act as a consultant, and show how the product can bring value and help clinically manage patients for whom the product is intended. I have a unique position in being a provider and having in-depth knowledge of the products I have worked with.

When you become an expert in a company's product and use it appropriately with your patients, and you have a solid understanding of the product, you might be asked to speak for the company and educate other providers on the clinical benefits and how you use the product in your practice. Speaking on behalf of these companies could lead to some extra cash on the side, and it is totally legit. If you work for a large hospital or company, you should check out their policies before agreeing to any speaking engagements. I spoke for a pacemaker company in the past, and it was a fantastic opportunity to educate doctors and staff on clinical guidelines for heart failure patients in addition to the benefits of the devices we spoke about. You could start saving for that little one's college sooner rather than later. I will have two in college as of this fall, and more of that money would have come in handy about now.

If you do research with your group and you need a company sponsorship of this research, you will need to contact their medical affairs division as the sales representatives are not involved in this process. You can however, reach out to them and get the medical affairs office information. They are not linked to the sales side of the company and will have a more clinical focus in nature. These companies are always looking to fund research projects with their products. So never hesitate to reach out and ask for funding.

There are so many good practice points to becoming a successful and productive PA. These are just the tip of the iceberg. You will find so many small nuances and tricks that keep you on your toes and on-track to being the most efficient, compassionate, and competent provider you can be. I know practicing some of these techniques will help you succeed. Don't be afraid to observe and seek out what your peers are doing to be successful. Steal their ideas and best practices. This is what I have done over the years to help be efficient, productive, and accomplished in my career. Purposefully pursue your way to greatness every day!

Chapter 8

Navigating Certification and Recertification

The more I live, the more I learn. The more I learn, the more I realize, the less I know.

—Michel Legrand

You'll never know everything about anything, especially something you love.

—Julia Child
Chef

I can just see all the eye-rolling and hear the sighs going on as you are dreading, even thinking about having to either certify or recertify. I mean really, haven't you already done enough? The answer is: Yes, you have! However, now you get to prove it again to yourself, the NCCPA, and every one you who is interested in your career—especially the pesky credentialing person in your office that starts bugging you three months before anything is even up for renewal.

In reality, you should have a good attitude toward credentialing. Our recertification sets us apart. Certification and recertification mean that we have standards. We must have standards for our profession. Not everyone who sets out to be a PA has what it takes. Having credentialing standards says every PA across the country, at any point in their career, knows the fundamentals and has a strong foundation in order to effectively practice medicine.

It means they don't want everyone who went to PA school to get to practice automatically. Did you have anyone in your class that was kind of questionable or just barely made it through? Did you wonder how in the world they continue to make it through every class? I had that person in my class. Being completely honest, I certainly didn't want her representing PAs. She was a disaster, and I'll just leave it at that, and I won't mention her idea of "professional attire." This is probably where my classmates would say it was me. Just kidding, maybe?

PA schools have an incentive for getting us through school. They want our tuition money, want to see us graduate, be successful, and serve our communities with care and expertise. Otherwise, it looks bad on them and their numbers. They need us to graduate and pass the exam as they usually advertise their graduation rate and their PANCE passing rate as well. It is in their best interest to help us get the best education and to pass our boards with flying colors. Remember, they are always on your side!

The reason we need certification is so that across the board, we know we all have what it takes to practice excellent medicine. Yes, you can see it as a pain to do and total anxiety-inducing experience. But in reality, it is for the good of our career. Not all PA schools are the same, and not everyone learns what they need to in order to practice medicine. After working with so many different types of providers and in so many different specialties, I have come to believe it is fantastic that we are nationally certified and that we have to recertify. Please do not cringe here.

Even though it is time-consuming and somewhat of a nuisance to do, it is a nice refresher to be up-to-date on best practices. For those who are focused and work in a specialty, it allows you an opportunity to bring you back to the basics of medicine. It helps keep in mind that we need to help our patients from a more holistic approach, taking into consideration every aspect of the patient's health.

The best providers I have ever worked with not only know just their specialty, but all aspects of medicine. You are treating the whole patient, not just the problem you see in front of you. You have to know other disease states and medication side effects that you don't regularly see or use, so that you can always keep them in the back of your mind as you evaluate your patients. Certifying and recertifying helps you establish and reestablish the foundation of your practice.

It is also helpful to refresh your memory to help friends and family who are always wanting that "quick question" answered. I have even had my docs I have worked with within specialty practice ask me medical questions that pertain to other areas of medicine. They know I have to stay current.

See recertification as an opportunity to reset and refocus and come back to basics. If you are interested in going into a new specialty or back to primary care, studying for recertification is an excellent time to hone-in on those skills that you will need for your new job. It will allow you to review the basics of that specialty so you will be ready to take on additional and more in-depth training prior to starting.

Your First Rodeo

For those of you who are certifying for the first time and taking the PANCE exam, you most likely are fresh out of school and probably are already well-prepared. Everything you have been learning is new in your mind, and you are just off your clinical rotations. Most likely, if you are just finishing up with your program, or are just finishing up school while you are taking the PANCE, you have no time to study at all. I suggest working on reviewing best practices, most common illnesses, and whatever area of medicine you do not feel as confident in. I did a bit more psychiatry than any other area, so I did not focus on reviewing any psychiatry. I didn't need to focus on this area. I was using it daily with family and friends, diagnosing all the crazy around me! Instead, I focused on endocrinology, and those areas that I still to this day, feel insecure about, along with the areas that I feel a little more bored with. Please don't ask me about metabolic acidosis. I only review and remember for test times, and then I promptly forget it.

If there is an inexpensive review course that your school offers, or something close by, you can certainly do these, but most likely, this is what you have been reviewing in class and clinical rotations the last several years. You may want to get one of the many review books available so you can look through these just to get familiar with how the test questions may look. Also, there are so many apps and websites available for review as well that may be helpful to you. If you happen to be in school, download these early. Even if you are unfamiliar with some of the terminology, guess and learn from the answers. Having at least a question a day roll in will keep you in the right mindset and will come in handy when it comes to testing time. There are even people on Instagram that post interactive exam questions several times a week. Find these people and follow them to keep up with a few questions here and there.

But my best advice, and in looking back on certification for the first time, this is when you will be on top of your game since you literally just went through training. And if you were paying attention and you learned during this time, you will do extremely well on the test! So do not stress out over it too much. At the end of training, everything will come together and making sense while you are in study mode, and on top of it. I think I was way more prepared for the PANCE exam than I have ever been for a PANRE exam.

Do not stress out if you do not pass it the first time and don't beat yourself up. Review the areas in which you did poorly, and then take the test over as soon as possible. You are not the first person who did not pass your first time. It happens. We all have bad days. Review test taking strategies and go out there and get it done the next time. Believe in yourself. You have what it takes!

Not Your First Rodeo

If you are taking the PANRE exam, again, this is an opportunity to keep up with medicine and current best practices. It is an excellent time for an overall review. Remember, PAs have a reputation for being well rounded in general medicine. I believe recertification is how we maintain this reputation.

NCCPA also has a program for an alternative to PANRE at this time. I recommend routinely visiting their website to see what all is new and available. If you are doing one of the newer tests they have available for specialties Certificate of Added Qualification (CAQS), this is a great way to show your knowledge set to your new practice. They currently have seven different CAQS. Remember, this is not a requirement, but it is an excellent way to have your resume stand out against any competition. A little interview tidbit—some newer studies have found that by doing these specialized tests, some PAs see increases in their salaries. It also shows your interest and commitment to that one area of medicine.

Keep Up With The Jones'

As a PA, we have many national and state requirements to keep up with for certification. Keeping up with these requirements will help you towards your certification and recertification as these requirements are primarily educational and help to further your career as a PA. Currently, the NCCPA requires 100 CME hours every two years, with at least 50 of these hours being Category 1, meaning formal training with conference CME, BLS/ACLS/PALS type courses, or reading and being tested over journal articles. All Category 1 hours must be approved by NCCPA through AAPA, ACCME, and AMA. And currently, self-assessment Category 1 CME is now worth an additional 50% per credit, and the first 20 PI-CME are now worth double.

You must log all of your hours before your recertification at the nccpa.net website. They will help you keep up with all of these hours, and some sites will automatically upload your credits for you. All of the requirements may change, so please look online regularly to be up to date with them. You will get emails from NCCPA. Make sure you add them to your contact list so these emails will not go to your spam account. These emails will remind you of what you are lacking. Just what we need is someone else telling us of how we are falling short, right? However, they are helpful and very nice reminders.

I can't tell you how many times I have been extremely close to the deadline of meeting the CME logging requirement. This last year, I had a goal to be done by October, and I think I finished by mid-November. Keep monthly goals and put them in your calendar on your phone to remind you. Time passes quickly, so you have to keep up with your hours. Don't be like me. I have looked for conferences in November where I can get all my hours in at one time, and all I could find were conferences in a not so fun location with, in my opinion, boring subject material. This could be a business suggestion for one of you; organize an interesting conference in November or December, in an easy to get-to location, where we could get in all of our hours. Send me an invite and a small royalty fee.

My suggestion is to keep a file folder or album within your phone's photos with all of your certificates. Then, every 3 to 4 months log onto NCCPA and record this information. This will help you when it's nearly time for your recertification deadline, and you are trying to cram your needed 27 hours of CME into a 24-hour time-period in-between Christmas and New Year's Eve. I promise I am going to take my own advice here too!

If you have the privilege to live in a big city, then you probably have lots of conferences of interest you can attend. Some organizations even put on CME conferences for free. If you have an interest in the courses being offered, then take advantage and go. If—like most—you have to pay for the conference, there is usually a discounted price for PAs.

I encourage you to attend conferences that have topics that you are interested in, even if it is not what field you may be practicing at the time. These conferences are great for CME and keeping up with clinical practice and guidelines. They are usually quite interesting and an easy way to network with physicians and PAs. In addition, I can't tell you the number of job offers I have been given at conferences by physicians I happened to sit next to. Once they see you that you are actively learning and are interested in the field, they will be eager to have you come to work with them! I even kept a letter from a gastroenterologist I met in the late 1990s asking me to move to Austin to join his practice.

You may find that once you get into a specialty, you gravitate towards conferences within your specialty. That is completely realistic. Not only will these conferences help you treat your patients better, but you can also bring back what you have learned and teach it to your peers. I have been to the ACC (American College of Cardiology), the AANS (American Association of Neurological Surgeons) and ACG (American College of Gastroenterology) annual conferences amongst many others. These are great conferences and have some up-to-date information and research trials that are extremely interesting and point towards the new direction of that specialty and how to practice. They may not necessarily help you prepare for your recertification exam as they are extremely detailed. So, once it is getting close to recertification time, you may want to attend conferences that offer a better overview of medicine to help you get prepared. There are also specialty allied health conferences as well that can be extremely valuable.

Review Courses

There are some excellent review courses you can attend that will help you prepare for your exam. One of the best I have heard about and have used each time I have recertified is CME Resources. It is an excellent course and well worth the money. Let's face it, with our hectic schedules, who has time and the discipline to study on their own? These courses are excellent for you to take time out of your otherwise too busy schedule. Yes, they will review Salter-Harris Fractures and all the other things you may have forgotten! You will review and take practice exams that will get you well prepared to walk in on exam day and do extremely well. They go over all general aspects of medicine that the PANCE and PANRE will test you over.

The practice exams will show where your weak spots are and help you get in exam-taking mode! If you choose a course because of its location and you think you will get to enjoy some of the scenery and night life—you should probably think again. These courses usually start early in the morning and go into the evening and have you take practice exams at night. They are mentally exhausting but well worth the effort! These courses can be a lot of fun and provide a place where you can meet other PAs, network for a new position, and catch up with your classmates.

If you are thinking about moving to a different city, you even may want to consider going to a conference in that city so you can network and see what opportunities are out there. I usually do a course a couple of months before my scheduled exam so that I can review the materials several times.

Journal Articles

Most of the journals we get have excellent and interesting review articles. Don't just throw them in a pile and wait for a rainy day to dig them out. When that rainy day comes, you will be taking a nap or doing something more fun than journal reading! Make an effort to read through at least one journal a week. I keep mine with my catalogs and will only look through a catalog if I have read the journal first. I know, I know, the games we must play to keep up with medicine! These journals are great and will keep you informed and up-to-date on current medical practice, and the PA specific journals are an excellent source of review leading up to recertification.

If you already know the information-don't read it, but if it is a subject you are interested in or not strong in, make an effort to go ahead and review it. You may not be using this information in your current job, but I guarantee it will come in handy for the exam, and for when that friend of a friend asks you over dinner what you know about Polycythemia Vera and all its complications, you will be ready. Yes, this is a true story. As I'm writing this part of the book, I happen to be in Mexico, and that was the question I got asked last night. My information for her was poor and fairly limited-telling me I should have read more of my journals! As a side note, when this happens, I often tell people I can get them to the appropriate website that will give them the information they need, or I can email them the information they are looking for at a later time.

As you read journals, make sure to log your CME hours. If you do testing and turn it in and get a certificate, it can be Category I CME. If you read and do not take tests, you may log this as Category II. Just keep up with how much you are reading to get accurate logging information for NCCPA.

Practice Tests

Taking practice tests and completing review questions are so important in doing well on the PANCE/PANRE. There are multiple apps now that have questions for review, and some of them offer you analytical data to help you know where your week points are so you can focus your studies. NCCPA also has practice tests for your review, and there are many review books that you can purchase to help you get ready for the exam. You need to know what you are getting yourself in for, so do not go into the testing situation without knowing what type of format the questions will be asked in.

The PANCE and PANRE are like any other standardized test, except you know this information, and you are already good at it! I know you are! And hopefully, you continue to be interested in medicine after going through school and being out in clinical practice. You will not know all the answers, and that's ok. You are not supposed to know all of them. Some of the questions are extremely difficult, and sometimes even experts in that particular specialty may not even know the answer. Just do your best and move on to the next question. Don't waste your time on something you have no clue about. Move on and focus on what you do know. If you have time in the end to review the difficult questions, go back, and review and reason your way through the question to come up with the best possible answer.

Exam Time

For all of you procrastinators, you already know medicine cannot be crammed into the night before your test. I'm sure if you are like me, lots of us have tried, and this leads only to anxiety and irritation with yourself! So don't do it!

Make sure you get a good night's sleep the day before the exam and make sure you give yourself plenty of time to get to the site before the test. Eat something, plan for traffic, and take a deep breath! You've got this, you have prepared, and you will kick some booty!

Testing Advice Itself

NCCPA.net is an excellent resource to answer all the technical questions you may have about certification and recertification. Their website has all the details and it is too much to cover in this book.

Take the test early enough so that you can have at least a couple of more tries before you lose your license. Your practice administrator will be after you. It would be extremely embarrassing and probably financially devastating not to be able to practice. You know you can do it, though, with proper planning, review, and early testing!

In summary, there are numerous resources available to you to help you prepare for the PANCE and PANRE. Keeping up with CME requirements, attending conferences, regularly using the review apps, and reading journal articles relevant to practicing medicine will be fundamental to your exam success. Know that there will be test questions meant to throw you for a loop. Don't get bogged down with these difficult and out of the ordinary questions. Focus on what you know, do your best, be prepared, and you will do an excellent job.

Chapter 9

Managing Difficult Issues

"The secret of success is learning how to use pain and pleasure instead of having pain and pleasure use you. If you do that, you're in control of your life. If you don't, life controls you."
—*Tony Robbins*

E veryone has a bad day every once in a while. No matter what field of medicine you go into as a PA, you will deal with difficulties, death, and poor outcomes. They may be with your patients. They may be with those you work with. They may be at home. Hopefully, they occur on an infrequent basis. Our character is defined on how we choose to handle the bad days, the sad days, and the "I don't feel like doing shit" days. Anyone can take the good days and be happy. What if we take the bad days and see them as opportunities to grow and better ourselves and those around us? Are we going to let circumstances or people control us?

I have spoken to my kids many times about drugs, friendships, and questionable situations that will arise throughout their life. I always say, "You have to know what you are going to do before you get there." It is not an *if* you will be in a situation, it is *when* you will be in one. If you already have the mindset of how you will best deal with negative situations and make the most out of them, then when the time comes, you will not be swayed by emotions that can be difficult to control.

I feel like I could have used this mindset to work through difficulties with my patients and those whom I work with way earlier in my career. I would get so frustrated and cringe and just get ridiculously worked up over the dumbest things. But once I chose to see these frustrations in a different light and have a plan of attack before I got involved, I handled things so much better. This is something that I still work on, but I am improving.

Could you choose to overlook and not get irritated when your physician double-checks to make sure you did something he asked of for the fourth time? Could you go into another room, away from the person sitting next to you who is chomping on their carrots like a horse, instead of cringing at each earth-shaking chomp? Could you laugh internally at Mrs. Parten while she is telling you about her crazy story she insists on telling you every time she comes in? Could you kindly respond to the nurse that asks you the same irrelevant question? You know these events are going to happen, don't you? When you change your mindset to adjust positively and see it as an opportunity to grow, it will help you deal with these issues so much better. You know things are going to come up. Life is not smooth. That would be boring. Ask yourself what you can learn, how you can grow and how you can serve others.

Hopefully, the bad days are few and far between, but for some of our fields, it is more frequent than we would like. We feel horrible for the patient and his/her family and what they have shared with us. We feel guilty as if there is a possibility that we could have done something wrong in how we treated someone. We sometimes feel fear and apprehension at the possibility of a lawsuit and peer reviews. My goodness, the list can go on and on. We put a lot of pressure on ourselves. We care so much, and we want the best outcomes for our patients, and we want the best environment to work within.

Risky Business

The worst day I have had thus far in my PA career is still vivid in my mind. It was with the unexpected death of one of my patients. He was highly active in his community, worked, and played golf several times a week. He was a patient, who if you saw him on your list of patients for the day you would be excited he was coming in. He was always pleasant, always a joy. He always made my day brighter. He had developed severe asymptomatic aortic stenosis, so I sent him to the cardiothoracic surgeon for evaluation. The surgeon recommended surgery and he reluctantly gave in and agreed.

I had made a note of the day of his surgery, and I kept checking his chart and his progress, waiting for any updates. Finally, I called the PA on service and learned that he had died the day of his surgery from multiple complications. I was devastated and felt horrible for him and his family. I wondered what did I do wrong, and if it was my fault that I sent him for further evaluation. I can still recall getting in the elevator and going to my office and sobbing. I adored that man and his family. It may seem simple and trite, as complications do occur, but when it's one of your favorite (yes, I do have my favorites) patients, it just makes you realize how precious life can be and how it can be gone in an instant.

There is a reason we go over risks, benefits, side effects, and alternatives to any medicine, procedure, and surgery. It's because all of them can and might happen and eventually will happen to one or some of your patients, and sometimes it's to the least suspecting ones. Each patient needs to make a well-informed decision. Never get complacent in explaining risks to patients. It may be your 257th time explaining the potential risks and benefits and alternatives to a recommended test, procedure, or surgery, but for your patient, it is the first time they are hearing about it.

Take your time, be thorough, and always ask if the patient has questions or concerns. Don't try to be in a rush to get out of the room. Sit down, look them in the eye, and let the patient know they are the most important item on the agenda!

Our job is truly a risky business. There are trials and difficulties that we often come across way too often. We must do a good job of preparing our patients and ourselves. We have to prepare them for any risk that may occur and we have to prepare ourselves that something may go wrong whether we sent them to surgery or we are performing the surgery. This is why it is so important to take care of your mental and physical health, as we have already mentioned. You have to be in the right frame of mind to optimally treat your patients and help them come to their best decision and you have to be prepared for anything that goes wrong once they make their decision.

Let Me Get This Right

You are your patient's best advocate! You have to look beyond the patient, the case, the medical condition in front of you, and help the patient and his/her family decide if whatever medicine, procedure, or surgery is right for them. Are they going to be better overall? Are they a good candidate? You can often hear me ask my patients, "What kind of job am I doing if I help you improve your quantity of life and I don't help you improve your quality of life?" Our job is to help the patient and his/her family comes to a decision that is best for them and their situation.

Several years ago, I was working with a patient who had severe coronary artery disease and needed a 3-vessel CABG. We had to postpone his surgery because he had a leg wound that had maggots living in it. And these were not at all the therapeutic ones. After several months, and who knows what kind of maggot treatment he had, they were eventually gone. Do they even teach you about getting rid of maggots in school? I think I missed that day or rotation completely. He was finally ready for his surgery, but after some conversation with the patient, I found out that his home environment was in disarray and his social situation was such that it was a major concern for his healing process. We first had to work in getting his living arrangements hygienic and in order before proceeding with his surgery and send him back to the house with the maggots and who knows what. He had a truckload of issues, and I did not do a thorough enough job upfront of getting the entire story, before recommending him to the cardiothoracic folks. Lesson learned yet again.

Make sure you are asking the right questions, especially with anyone who you are concerned about their living conditions and their mental conditions as well. There can be way more to the story than you even realize. Especially asking, is this the right procedure or surgery for you at this time?

Are you able to take care of yourself at home? Or who is going to help you when you get home? And in some cases, do you have a home to go back to?

Who is going to drive you home after your surgery/procedure?

Who helps you with your medications? Are you going to remember to take a pill three or four times a day?

Who is going to take care of you after your surgery? Is this a situation like my ex-husband who brought me home after outpatient surgery, dropped me off and went back to work for the day and then went out of town the next morning for the weekend?

Are there any other medical conditions we need to know about that might hinder this treatment/surgery/procedure?

Do you realize you will have a lifting restriction of less than 10 pounds for several months after surgery? This is important for those patients who work and cannot return to work on light duty and may not be able to afford the time off.

Understand your patients, educate, and help them come to a conclusion that is best for their outcome. I have seen circumstances far too often where patients did not clearly understand how much pain they would be in after their surgeries. They had no clue as to the recovery and restrictions they would need to abide by.

What's Your Opinion?

Frequently our patients ask for our opinion. I realize that we get paid to give our professional advice. We educate our patients on risks, benefits, alternatives, side effects, and have that whole laundry list of disclaimers after we speak about any therapy. But sometimes patients want to know what we would do if we, or one of our loved ones, were in their situation. Sometimes giving an opinion is very straightforward, and other times it can be very difficult just to come out and say what you feel is right. I often tell my patients and have heard other providers do the same, "If you were my dad or brother, I would _____" fill in the blank with your recommendations.

One day while in the cardiology clinic, I got a call from one of the ICU attendings, asking if I could speak to one of the patient's wives about turning off his ICD (Implantable Cardioverter Defibrillator) as they did not want it to shock him since he had such a poor prognosis. I had known the patient and his wife for years, as I had followed him for his heart failure. We had managed his ICD, and I got to know him very well during our appointments. When I went upstairs to see him, his wife met me at his door and collapsed, crying into my arms and telling me that she just could not decide without my opinion first. I began crying with her because we both loved him so very much. What a huge honor it is to help our patients and their families through situations like this! A device feature recommended for its life-saving capabilities is now being turned off so that the patient can die as peacefully as possible.

Always look at the patient and everything that is going on with them as a whole. Just because we can do something, doesn't mean we should. You may criticize this thought, but I think it is important to know your patients' long term wishes and desires. Work with your patients and their families to get them involved with social workers, support group services, and other available resources to help them through difficult situations. Our patients deserve to live and die with dignity and respect, and it is our job to help them accomplish this by educating them to the best of our ability.

You can't go wrong by always keeping the patient and their well-being at the forefront of everything you do. Well, at least you can live with yourself if you always keep your patient first.

There will be difficult days and tough decisions as you go through your career as a PA. Knowing that you keep up with best practices in medicine, helping your patients make the right decisions by giving them as much information as possible, and doing your best every single day, will help you through these times and ensure the best possible outcome. Take a deep breath. You've got this!

Legal Eagles

Unfortunately, I've come to see every patient that I care for as a potential lawsuit. For some reason, this phrase just stuck with me for my entire career. I know no one wants to talk about lawsuits, and we are all scared of them, but it is something to keep in mind. I already mentioned the horror of being named in a lawsuit. I was served papers at my home and had to review tons of medical records and go by myself to downtown Houston for a deposition. I still carry the paperwork of the dismissal of any wrongdoing on my part to every single job I have taken since. This is because everyone wants to know if you have even been named in a suit. And you know what? It totally sucks, but I made it through, and I am just fine.

Lawsuits happen in medicine. It is why we have insurance, and I promise you, you will get through it! Maybe some tears, embarrassment, and WTF moments, but you will make it through. Do not go through anything like this alone. Do not isolate yourself in shame or embarrassment. Call one of your PA friends. Talk to them and let them be there for you as you go through anything like this. You would never want your colleagues to go through this. You would completely be there for them if they needed you. Allow them to be there for you in this time. If you have to go to court or go to a deposition, ask someone to go with you.

We Are In This Together

Practicing medicine can be extremely stressful. You will have difficulties that can surround you and feel like they are swallowing you up. This is why it is so important to take care and be kind to yourself, as we have spoken about throughout this book. If you are struggling with any depression or thoughts of suicide, please get help immediately. You are not alone.
Speak to someone, anyone. You would be more than willing to drop anything if someone came to you with a concern. You would not be judgmental, you would want to help. Others are willing to do the same for you, but you have to let someone know. Tell a friend, family member, or someone in your office.

Call a fellow PA. Being a physician assistant means you are part of a huge family; a family who cares about you and wants the best for you. Do not suffer alone. Get help when you need it.

Chapter 10

The Importance of Developing Business Skills In Your Practice Setting

Your most unhappy customers are your greatest source of learning.

—Bill Gates

"Girls like guys with skills."

—Napoleon Dynamite

So many of us go to PA school, and we just want to get done, get a great job making a good income to support our spending habits, and get some recognition along the way from our patients and our coworkers. It is important to realize that medicine is a business and to be a purposeful PA, you have got to grow your skills as a savvy business professional. Good PAs show up to work every day, do their job and leave for the day, great PAs look to see how they can grow their practice or hospital's business and give the best most up-to-date care available to their patients. You will find that there are many improvements that you can suggest. If you are willing to complain, you must be willing to do something about it. Come up with a plan that has actionable solutions to help contribute to growth, efficiency, and patient care.

Coding For Dollars

How can you grow your business for your company or group? Well, you can begin by working on learning how to properly code for the services you provide. If you are your practice's or hospital's first PA, they are not necessarily going to know how to bill for your services. Do your homework and research coding information. Your practice or hospital will have a coder. Sit down with this individual and work with them, so they know how to bill for your services effectively and efficiently.

I think one of the best things you can do is attend a coding class in your specialty. Again, this may be something you may have to pay for out of pocket but do it. Search for any online coding classes and take what you can. Know what you are worth and help your practice be aware of how and where to utilize your strengths. This information will also be helpful when your evaluation comes up. You can know exactly how much money you have brought in for your practice and what you are worth. There is nothing wrong with keeping track of this information. I guarantee that all of the doctors you are working with are doing it. They need that commission check to keep rolling in. Keep a notes section on your phone daily or weekly so you can keep up. You should know how valuable you are in any area you are in.

If within your specialty, you work with representatives from medical device companies within the operating room or something similar, realize that they have reimbursement specialists that can help you with coding as well. Have them get you in contact with these specialists who can walk you through the ins and outs of their devices. It's in their interest to help you understand so you have no confusion about coding for, implanting, and using their products.

The Profit Practice

Having a keen sense of running a business is a practice I would highly recommend. I had the opportunity to audit some business classes when my children's father was attending Northwestern to get his MBA. Not only did I learn a lot about business from speaking to him about what his classes were teaching him, but I also sat in on a negotiation class that has helped me in every job offer I have negotiated for since that time. I had no idea how much of an interest in business I had until I started learning more. I had never really thought of any practice I was a part of as a money-making business until then. I only focused on the patient aspect of medicine. But truly, to treat patients well, you must run a hospital and/or practice that is both ethical and profitable.

Take an interest in your practice, learn from those around you, and seek opportunities to grow your business skills, then speak up and add value to your practice. Sit with the schedulers and understand your appointment template. Look to see how you can gain efficiency. If you are getting paid on how many patients you see per day, this can be a helpful practice to see how you can see patients as effectively and efficiently as possible. Once your coworkers and physicians know that you are taking an interest, it might encourage them to do so as well. And when you come up with some time-saving or better yet money-saving ideas, they will see you as even more of an asset than before.

Supply Chain

Understand the supply ordering process for all the things you do on a daily basis. Someone has to order the Band-Aids and the paper for the tables and the toilet paper for the office. Find ways to help make the ordering process appropriate and more efficient.

Learn the staffing and hiring process if you are interested and have time. Understand the importance of cross-training staff for coverage. Each person will be on vacation or sick and it is nice if everyone around can pitch in and do the other one's job to help out. Train each individual for their job and make sure they have the customer service skillset they need to go above and beyond with patient care. Even if it isn't part of your regular job, volunteer to help train new staff that you will be working with on a regular basis. It will be so nice for them to have your encouragement and it gives you an opportunity to make sure they are being trained in the ways of the practice that will be beneficial to both you and your patients.

If you are in a hospital setting, go to town halls and network with those in leadership. Sometimes they will ask you to be a part of different committees within the hospital. You can even volunteer to help. You have so much value to add. I guarantee that you see things in a light other people around you do not. They need people like you to offer your insight and great ideas.

By always keeping the patient in mind at every turn and understanding different avenues of the inter-office working environment, and adding value to the process where you can, you will be more than beneficial to your staff and your practice.

Improve The Flow

Seek to find more efficient ways to see patients. Make the flow easier, and your daily office operations smoother. Don't be afraid to offer suggestions and put forward proposals to make things better for your practice. This is how change works. Be the voice of change. Do not just complain, but seek to understand, and provide helpful solutions.

Get Verified

If you are in surgery, please know how important it is for your patient to show up. This little break might be nice for you and give you a little breather for the day, but if you don't have office staff to call and confirm times and surgeries, and your patients do not show up, this is a loss of revenue. It also takes away a spot for someone else who might have to wait longer for their surgery.

Confirming appointments and surgeries is crucial. Lord, my hair salon knows when my grays are coming in. They call me, text me and email me starting three days before my appointment and up until the morning of my appointment. It doesn't matter if I confirmed each and every time or even made the appointment the day before. They want to make sure that I am coming in because they depend on that income for them and their family.

Self-Education

Take a few business classes or listen to podcasts or listen to books while commuting to work. Take some tips and tricks from experts on how to make your practice productive, marketable, and efficient in all areas. Occasionally at the larger conferences, they will have business practice sessions that are specific to your specialty, and these talks can be helpful for you as well. This information will also help you understand your practice model and how and why your business runs the way it does. Since we don't get much business training in school, it is up to us to have a foundational understanding of the practice business model we are employed by.

Serve With A Smile

I also believe in being very customer service oriented and focused. Yes, you are there to see patients and care for them. But do you know what they experience? Your goal shouldn't just be to take care of the patient in front of you. Make sure your patients have a fantastic and welcoming experience no matter where in the clinic or hospital setting they are.

After many visits to the gynecologist I have been seeing for years here in Kansas City, I finally got the courage to tell him that his front office staff was very rude. I call for an appointment—they are rude. I call to get results—they are rude. I come to the appointment—they are rude, not even glancing my way, too busy on Facebook and social media. I'm so sorry that I have inconvenienced you by thinking that you were going to be doing your job today and do it courteously. Seriously? I simply told him that I thought he and his nurse were great, but I did not like working with his other staff. He was very apologetic and thanked me for giving him feedback because many patients would not so.

Ok, call me Karen like my kids do. It's ok. I am an improver and an informer, and I expect to be treated well. I also want people to be aware of what they might be missing. I would definitely want to know if someone employed by me was treating my customers poorly. And he was missing the point that he and his partners were letting a bunch of bitches run his front office. I am sure that I had no part at all in changing his impolite office staff, but it has been several years now, and I can't tell you what a positive change I see. They are polite, nice, and always kind to everyone who walks in. It makes going to the gynecologist and being poked and prodded better if at least the office staff is helpful and friendly.

Make sure you ask your patients what their impression is. How have they been treated? How was their appointment, check-in, and rooming experience? How were the staff that put your IV in or got you ready for your procedure? How are things going? How up to date are the magazines in the front office? Encourage your practice to do surveys. Ask about the entire experience the patient may have. Call in yourself and see how long it takes to speak with a real person. Sit in the front lobby and to see where the cobwebs are and how old and dirty the magazines are. Is this a place where you would like to come as a patient? If the answer is no, strive to make the changes you want to see.

You have to realize that getting a patient to come to see you once or twice is usually easy. Make sure you are setting yourself apart by being an office where the patients come back and don't doctor shop. Medicine is competitive. Be unique. Make sure you set your patients up for the best experience to keep them coming back and referring their friends. My kids saw an orthodontist when they were young, who had the coolest office with up-to-date technology and modern decor. They loved going because it was fancy, and the staff made them feel special every time they walked in. If you have the ability to make these kinds of changes, do so and if you think you don't have the ability, it never hurts to ask to see what kind of changes can be made.

Be A Boss

These are just a few aspects of hospital and clinical practice. You will be exposed to so much more and be given the opportunity to learn about business in different and unique ways. I wish I had educated myself about the business of medicine from the start of my career. I might have even established my own practice and had the doctors working for me. There are NP's and PAs out there with their own practices and urgent care clinics. They have been extremely successful with this. They have taken time to learn that medicine is a business and one where it can be quite lucrative.

In Missouri and several other states, doctors have opened and own ambulatory surgery centers. Not only are they getting paid on the surgery they perform, but they are also getting paid on the surgery center fee as well. They have found a money-making business model that works for them. You can do the same if you are creative, have an interest, and follow the rules, laws, and regulations.

Learning the foundational business model of your practice can be helpful, and make you and your practice more efficient. It can save time, money, and make caring for patients more streamlined and more customer-friendly. We want our patients—or at least the majority of them—to feel as welcome, comfortable, and relaxed as possible from the moment they walk in the door, all the way through working with our billing department for the EOBs and bills they get and have difficulty understanding. This is one of the most important parts to having patients returning to your office, and having those patients refer their friends and family to you. This is job security and longevity.

Chapter 11

Exploring Additional Pathways as a Physician Assistant

"Your work is going to fill a large part of your life, and the only way to be truly satisfied is to do what you believe is great work. And the only way to do great work is to love what you do. If you haven't found it yet, keep looking. Don't settle. As with all matters of the heart, you'll know when you find it."

—*Steve Jobs*

Being a physician assistant can be challenging in and of itself. There are always new things to learn. New medicines, procedures, research, journals, and new conferences are always available. There are billing challenges and coding headaches and all types of obstacles we face in being a PA. Doing the same thing day in and day out can become quite tedious. We need to challenge ourselves in our careers. Move forward. Grow. Don't be complacent.

Specialty Shop

Having been a physician assistant for 24 years now, I have been in four different specialties. This continually creates a new challenge by learning a new specialty and it definitely keeps me on my toes. Not that I have mastered all of them, but it has been exciting and difficult at the same time. So I would encourage you to consider changing specialties if you're bored, and it seems like the medicine you are practicing is monotonous. Starting in a new specialty is like starting a new career. There are cool new procedures and instruments and medicines. It's all bright and shiny and new and can be so much fun. And there are so many awesome opportunities out there for you.

C-Suite Opportunities

Consider going into administration. There are many physician assistants out there who represent our profession well by leading with their administrative skills. If you're in a large clinic, you could certainly be your practice administrator. If you do not feel you have the skills for this, you could consider getting an MBA or health care administration degree and go on to become a CEO of a healthcare company, hospital, or insurance company. We need physician assistants to do things like this so that we have representation in these areas.

You can look for opportunities within your own organization in your current position. Consider teaching within the organization. If you're in a big healthcare practice, look for opportunities to train staff, your peers, and ancillary staff. Your staff needs to understand why we make some of the decisions we make, like why patients need certain procedures or educate them on some of the common diseases that you treat in your office. When everybody is knowledgeable about what is going on, this makes for better patient care. Encourage and educate those around you. It will also build relationships with your staff, and they will have even more respect for you for taking an interest in their education.

Guest of Honor

You can also look for guest speaker opportunities with pharmaceutical companies, device companies, and local charitable organizations such as the American Red Cross and American Heart Association. Volunteer for speaking engagements within your community. Some of the pharmaceutical and device companies also offer a stipend for guest speakers. In addition, these engagements can lead to national speaking opportunities. I have volunteered within my hospital and the Veteran's Association of Physician Assistants and have had the honor of speaking at several national meetings.

Raise Your Hand

Volunteerism is a great networking opportunity and helps solidify your expertise within your field and can even lead to more speaking engagements. As one of my friends says, "Never miss an opportunity to address an audience!" Take advantage of these engagements to represent your specialty, your profession, and give back to your community. I'd rather the people around me be on the same page as I am and understand as best as possible the disease states we discuss. While speaking with patients in the community and educating them and their family members, realize that this can be a marketing opportunity for you and your practice.

Back To School

Consider becoming a faculty member or being a preceptor for local physician assistant schools. I don't think I had the best preceptor. She was a bit grumpy, seemingly overworked, and just not what I was hoping for in giving me the best advice and teaching. I vowed to become a preceptor when possible and make a difference for the students I worked with. I have worked with several PA schools in different cities and have enjoyed working with every student. I encourage you to call your nearest PA school up and offer your help. These schools don't always know if you would be interested in volunteering your time, so why not reach out to them.

Our schools need faculty and preceptors who are interested in our students and the future of our profession. This is a great opportunity for you to perfect your physical diagnosis skills as well as teach others. These students require your wisdom and encouragement to help build a firm foundation in which to practice medicine. PA students need good leaders to follow and emulate.

Legal Pad

When I first got out of training, I did contract work for a law firm that defended against medical malpractice within nursing homes. They would send me patient charts in which I would review the entire chart looking to find any issues within the chart that were not consistent or alarming. I would then provide an objective report of my findings. This would be quite helpful for the law firm to evaluate the type of care the patient received and if there was any negligence involved.

This type of work is quite—ok extremely—tedious, but very interesting and can be quite helpful to the firm. It feels like being a private investigator in the chart and can be kind of fun. It definitely reminds you of the importance of documentation in every detail of patient care. Besides, this type of contract work pays very well. It was nice to have some extra spending cash. If you are interested, search out medical law firms to work with or ask any of your lawyer friends that you have in your network.

Out Of The Box

If you get a little tired of being a physician assistant, you can also look for other opportunities where your clinical background will be highly valued.

Many physician assistants go back to medical school. If you have the desire and the time, just do it and don't look back later and wish you would have. You will be the most qualified candidate and smartest first year ever!

PAs also become pharmaceutical, medical device representatives, clinical specialists, clinical educators, clinical consultants, and medical science liaisons. I am not encouraging you to leave your profession, but there are opportunities where your background and expertise can be highly valued and well utilized. Having been in this area and working in sales, my managers and team have valued my clinical knowledge and insight. And I have enjoyed the opportunity to educate the physicians, PAs and NPs on amazing products and how they can benefit some of their patients.

Surprisingly, some of these roles will come with a nice salary increase and an incentive compensation plan where you can be rewarded for your hard work. You will find there are many needs in medicine, and you may come up with an idea for a device, software, or service that will lead you into your own start-up company. This is a dream of mine. I would love to start my company and be my own boss and do something completely disruptive in medicine to make life better for patients. I'm still working on ideas. My current one is that my husband and I launched a podcast for patients called The Well-Informed Patient Podcast where we interview experts and patients on life-changing medical devices, laboratory testing, and therapeutics that are not always offered by providers.

What ideas do you have that you could turn into a company for change and positivity? I encourage you to take action and make it happen. Medicine needs people like you to start companies that will positively impact our world. Heck, start it in your garage in your spare time, like Earl Bakken, the founder of Medtronic.

Madam President

Our profession needs excellent representation. Consider running for a state or national office position. There are multiple professional PA organizations. I encourage you to serve our profession.

If you are a PA, you are a leader. Have the confidence in yourself to know that you can run any organization and contribute your valuable opinion. Within the next 10 to 15 years, our career will continue to grow and expand. There will be multiple changes, and you have an opportunity to become a leader within your community and your profession and help lead the direction of our profession. I have found that when I am about to complain about a situation, I must be willing to step up and lead the positive changes. You have everything it takes to step forward and lead our profession.

If not you, then who?

The Happy Choice

Regardless of how long you stay in your current position, which specialty of medicine you practice, or where you end up, choose to be happy. It has taken many years of my life to realize that happiness is a choice. There will always be disappointments, challenges, and obstacles to overcome. Choose to be content. You cannot help what others do, but you can be responsible for how you act and your attitude.

When you have a great attitude and are happy about life, it helps others be encouraged to be the same. Please, please, please don't stay in any job that you hate and dread coming to every day. If you are being mistreated or you do not like what you are doing, it is up to you to change your circumstance. I truly believe in the statement that insanity is doing the same thing over and over again and expecting a different outcome. You cannot go to work over and over again and expect work to change. It will not. Life is incredibly too short to be miserable. Complaining won't change your circumstances. You have to do something for things to change. Nobody is going to come up to you and say, "Are you not happy in your job? Let me find you a better one." No, it is your responsibility. Refuse to be the victim. You spend way too much time at work not to be happy. You can definitely find a better work environment. I promise you.

Do What You Are Good At

I believe you will be told what you are good at by those around you. You may not think you are good at something, but when you are repetitively told something over and over and by different individuals, listen to them.

I am continuously told I am a really good encourager and a great teacher. It's true, I love to teach and educate those around me. I even do it to people who don't solicit my opinion. Yes, I know it's a fault, but when you give patients your advice all day every day, this just transfers over to every other aspect of your life. These are the things I love to do!

Along your career path, you will be encouraged to what you are good at… follow that path! Find an area where you can do what you excel in and continue developing that skill. You will not be unsatisfied by doing what you love and what you are good at.

Be All That You Are Meant To Be

I love being a PA, and I love our profession and hate to see good PAs leave, but you have to do what you are called to do. Who cares if you change your occupation or go outside of being a PA? Life is too short to put up with the same job that you dislike every day.

God has put it on my heart to do something beyond what I was doing, and writing this book is the first thing. Continue to seek your heart, to strive for the best in your life, and share your passion and your gifts with those around you. Do what you love and grow your best career path for you.

Live in the here and now. Be present and know that you are a PA by no mistake. You are called to be where you are for a reason and purpose. You have every bit of what it takes. You have passion, drive, and compassion. You never stop learning. You are purposeful in all that you do, and you do it to the best of your ability!

Post Script

I want to thank you for taking time to read this book. I truly believe you are meant for so much more than mediocre. The PA profession is a platform for you to make a difference in so many lives from right where you are. You are a leader and you will make a difference in this society.

I started this book in late 2012, wrote the outline in a day and wrote 50% of it fairly quickly and then put it on the shelf until January of 2020. I kept feeling a calling to write this and get it out to you. It was a really long time coming but I made a commitment in January to get it done and then COVID came and left me without a job in April of 2020, so I had plenty of time to get it done. I have called, written, and emailed publishers to no avail and have chosen to self-publish this because I know we all need encouragement and pointers in our career.

I hope this book is helpful for you and points you in a positive direction to always be purpose-driven in your life and in your career. You got this!

Acknowledgments

First of all, I would like to thank the PA profession for giving me a fantastic career. To be honest, I need to thank everything in my life, both good and bad. Good tells us, you got this! Bad is what makes us and gives us perseverance.

I am very thankful for so many people. I could not have done this without my husband Jonathan who came along way too late in my life, but has been a constant cheerleader and has allowed me to talk incessantly about my goals and getting this book in your hands.

I am thankful for my two children, Miles and Connor. They have made me a better person and allowed me to live childhood all over again and in so much of a fun way. You are both awesome and I love being your mom more than anything. I like turtles.

I am thankful to Sandy Epperson, my counselor who has helped me grow in confidence and wisdom over the last 16 years. She helped me see that I am enough all by myself and everything else is icing!

Thank you to my mom, my dad, and my sister who made me the strong person I am today and have taught me how to persevere.

I am forever grateful for my Aunt Nancy and Uncle Dee who have always encouraged me and given me wisdom and totally honest guidance.

I am ever so thankful to so many of the doctors, PAs and staff members that I have worked with in my profession. Dr. James Wolter taught me to be calm in a storm, Dr. Michael Liston taught me everything he knows about cardiology and answered every single page and text and call, Dr. Peter Schwarz, gave me my first PA job and encouraged me to keep learning and growing and to get my butt to grand rounds at UT at 7am in the mornings. I am always in awe of Magdalene Akanji, my best VA PA neurosurgery friend who encouraged me to work out, eat better, take life less seriously, and to make money in my sleep.

I am thankful to my sweet friends Cheryl, James, and Kim who encouraged me to get this thing done and have taught me lots of life lessons; mainly about how to live well!

I owe my career path at BCM to Carl Fasser, who answered my call when I didn't get in to PA school the first time I tried and was so kind and gave me suggestions of what to do for the next year. He was a fantastic PA school director and I truly believe, The Father of the PA profession!

I love the patients I have been able to serve and who have given me amazing life lessons and have been so kind to share their life with me and trust me with their care; any patient names mentioned in this book have been changed to protect them.

I am built from Christian and self-help books like Beth Moore, Joel Osteen, Tony Robbins, Gary Chapman, Henry Cloud, Shad Helmstetter and the list goes on.

Thank you, my fellow PAs and those just interested in the profession who inspired me to write this book. I know you will do so well out there!

Made in United States
Troutdale, OR
07/17/2024

21276913R00097